MRCP PART 2
REVISION BOOK

D0755392

MRCP PART 2
REVISION BOOK

Compiled and edited by
EVA LESTER, MBBS MRC Path
Consultant Chemical Pathologist, North Middlesex Hospital, London.

Foreword by
I. D. RAMSAY, MD FRCP
Consultant Physician, North Middlesex Hospital, London.

PASTEST SERVICE
Hemel Hempstead
Hertfordshire
England

First published 1982

British Library Cataloguing in Publication Data
MRCP Part 2 revision book
1. Pathology—Problems, exercises, etc.
1. Lester, Eva
616'.0076   RB119
ISBN 0 906896 08 8

Phototypeset and Printed by Martin's of Berwick.

CONTENTS

FOREWORD

This book has been compiled by doctors teaching on the North Middlesex MRCP Part II course and has been put together and edited by Dr. Eva Lester. The questions contained in it reproduce, as far as possible, the sort of questions which are encountered in the actual examination. The most profitable way of using this book is to go through the questions and answer them within the given time limits. This will give you practice in coming to quick decisions about the correct answers. The answers can then be looked up and thought about in a more leisurely manner.

It should be emphasised that this book is only a practice run-through for the examination. It does not set out to teach internal medicine. You can only learn medicine by seeing and examining a wide variety of patients, paying special attention to areas of difficulty such as neurology. This will not only help you with slide recognition, data interpretation and the "grey" cases but will stand you in good stead for the clinicals. Practice doing previously unseen long cases on firms other than your own and presenting them to the consultant on his ward round as you would to the examiners in the M.R.C.P. Attend ward rounds other than your own consultant's and ask to do short cases.

Do not fail yourself! You may antagonise some examiners by appearing excessively hirsute or eccentrically dressed. It is worth-while buying (or even hiring) a sober suit, shirt, tie and shoes and paying a visit to the barber. After all, you can always re-grow the flowing locks and beard after you have passed the exam. Be polite to the patients. Introduce yourself and ask permission to examine them. Thank them at the end and help them with their night clothes and tuck in the sheets and blankets. That will at least show that you are a courteous and considerate doctor.

If, during an interrogation on short or long cases, you realise you have said something foolish, you should immediately retract it and say that it is wrong. Most examiners will realise that it was caused by nervousness and will not penalise you too heavily. If you do not know something it is best to say so, rather than to blurt out something wrong, which you may be tempted to justify (to your cost).

Lastly, if the examiners get on to a subject about which you know quite a lot, do not make this readily apparent by going into an exhaustive monologue about it. Allow the examiners to ask you several questions about the subject so that they do not immediately move on to another subject of which you may be totally ignorant.

Ian Ramsay MD FRCP
Clinical Tutor and organiser of the
North Middlesex Part II Course.

INTRODUCTION

The MRCP Part II written examination consists of three sections.

Case histories. There are four compulsory questions to be answered in 55 minutes. Each is a case history with the results of the physical examination. The questions are designed to test skill in diagnosis, planning of investigations and management. You need to have both good background knowledge and the ability to think straight to give what is not necessarily the only "correct" answer but the best answer.

Data Interpretation. There are 10 sets of data to be interpreted in 45 minutes. There is usually a very short clinical description followed by the results of biochemical or haematological laboratory tests, electrocardiograms, lung function tests or cardiac catheter studies. You are expected to know the normal ranges for those constituents which you regularly ask to be measured and where the methods used by different laboratories are sufficiently standardised to give a (more-or-less) universal range. They are only quoted in the question when the results of more exotic tests are included.

Projected material. The examination paper contains 20 compulsory questions each based on a slide or a pair of slides projected in a lecture theatre for 2 minutes. A bell rings half a minute before each slide changes. You are asked to write short answers in the question and answer book which is provided. The slides are prepared from clinical and retinal photographs, radiographs, including arteriograms, myelograms and barium studies. There may be a blood film, bone marrow aspirate or occasionally a histological slide. Project facilities are excellent and the theatre is arranged so that there is a good view of the screen from all seats.

The aim of this book is to provide practice in all sections. It is arranged in three parts, the first with 30 case histories, the second with 66 data interpretation questions, and the third with 64 colour plates as a more convenient way of reproducing the projected material in the examination than by providing sets of slides which require you to find your own projection facilities. Finally there are practice case history and data interpretation examinations so that you can test your ability to answer questions within the correct timespan.

Eva Lester

CONTRIBUTORS

P. Burnett   MRACP
Caroline Dunn   MRCP
Anita Harding   MRCP
T. O. Kumaran   Ph.D. MRCP MRC Path
J. H. Parr   MRCP
I. D. Ramsay   MD FRCP
P. Ranmuthu   MRCP
Jeanne Reeve   FRC Path
F. J. Woodroffe   M.Sc. FRCP
I. D. Woolf MA MRCP

TABLE OF NORMAL RANGES

CHEMICAL PATHOLOGY

Plasma or serum constituent		Range
Alkaline phosphatase		30-115 iu/l
Amylase		70-300 iu/l
Aspartate transaminase		⟨ 40 iu/l
Bicarbonate		24-32 mmol/l
Bilirubin		⟨ 17 micromol/l
Calcium		2.1-2.6 mmol/l
Chloride		95-105 mmol/l
Cholesterol		⟨ 5.7 mmol/l
Complement C3		1.0-2.0 g/l
Cortisol	Midnight	80-320 nmol/l
	9 a.m.	280-700 nmol/l
Gamma glutamyl transferase	Men	6-28 iu/l
	Women	4-18 iu/l
Glucose (fasting)		3.5-6.5 mmol/l
Lactate		1.0-1.8 mmol/l
Magnesium		0.7-1.9 mmol/l
Osmolality		275-295 mmol/kg
pH		7.35-7.45
PCO_2		35-45 mm Hg (4.6-6.0 kPa)
PO_2		95-105 mm Hg (12.6-14.0 kPa)
Phosphate (inorganic)		0.8-1.4 mmol/l
Potassium		3.5-5.0 mmol/l
Prolactin		360 mU/l
Protein Total		62-82 g/l
Albumin		35-50 g/l
Sodium		136-148 mmol/l
Total Thyroxine		55-160 nmol/l
TSH		⟨ 10 mU/l
Triglyceride		⟨ 1.7 mmol/l
Urea		2.5-6.5 mmol/l
Uric Acid		0.1-0.4 mmol/l

TABLE OF NORMAL RANGES

HAEMATOLOGY

Haemoglobin	Men	13.5-18.0 g/dl
	Women	11.5-16.5 g/dl
Red cell count	Men	4.5-6.5 × 10^{12}/1
	Women	3.8-5.8 × 10^{12}/1
Packed cell volume	Men	0.40-0.54
	Women	0.37-0.47
Mean corpuscular haemoglobin		27-32 pg
Mean corpuscular volume		77-93 fl
Mean corpuscular haemoglobin concentration		31-35 g/dl
Reticulocyte count		0.2-2.0%

White blood cell count		
	Total	4.0-11.0 × 10^9/1
	Neutrophils	2.0-7.5 × 10^9/1
	Lymphocytes	1.5-4.0 × 10^9/1
	Monocytes	0.2-0.8 × 10^9/1
	Eosinophils	0.04-0.4 × 10^9/1
	Basophils	Up to 0.1 × 10^9/1

Platelets		150-400 × 10^9/1
Serum vitamin B12		160-925 ng/1
Serum folate		3-20 µg/1
Red cell folate		160-640 µg/1
Serum iron	Men	14-32 micromol/1
	Women	10-30 micromol/1
Total iron binding capacity		50-80 micromol/1
Transferrin		2.0-4.0 g/l

handwritten notes: ie 1/3 saturated; ~ 18; ~ 54

x

CASE HISTORIES

1. A 24 year old woman was admitted complaining of pain in the lower back radiating down the left leg and some associated pain in the left hip. In addition she was complaining of a painful swollen right knee.
    There was a past history of pleurisy 6 years earlier.
    On examination a pale thin woman with under-developed upper extremities. C.N.S. Absent pulses noted in the left arm. Femorals and all lower limb pulses easily palpable. Fundi normal. Joints—effusion right knee which was warm and tender. Limitation of all movements at the left hip. Reduced straight leg raising on left.

    Investigations:

    Hb 12.6 g/dl
    WBC 8.9 × 10⁹/1
    ESR 57 mm/hr
    Chest X-ray normal
    X-ray pelvis—some sclerosis of both sacro-iliac joints. Left hip normal
    R.A. Latex test. Negative
    LE cells not seen

    Questions:
    1. What is the diagnosis?
    2. What investigation would confirm it?
    3. What is the treatment for this condition?

Answers overleaf

1. 1. Takayashu's arteriopathy.
2. Aortography.
3. Corticosteroids, with or without anticoagulants.

2. A 29 year old male was admitted as an emergency with a five
day history of colicky central abdominal pain radiating to the
epigastrium and right hypochondrium associated with dyspepsia
and vomiting. Diarrhoea at onset possibly related to the
ingestion of Milk of Magnesia as a remedy for indigestion.
The past medical history included an appendectomy in 1970.
On examination temperature 38.2°C. pulse 104/min regular,
blood pressure 130/80 mm/Hg, no cardiac murmurs, lungs
clear, abdomen marked tenderness in the epigastrim with
guarding and rebound tenderness, no masses palpable, bowel
sounds intact, grid iron appendectomy scar.

Investigations:

Hb 13.2 g/dl
WBC 7.1 × 10⁹/1 (83% neutrophils)
Chest X-ray normal
Plain X-ray of abdomen, erect and supine, no abnormalities
    detected
Serum amylase 196 iu/l
Plasma urea 2.9 mmol/l
Electrolytes normal

Progress and treatment. He was admitted for observation and
for the next four days showed a swinging pyrexia reaching a
peak of 39.5°C. He continued to complain of severe epigastric
tenderness and on examination four days after his initial
admission marked rebound tenderness was again demonstrable.
Repeat serum amylase was 100 iu/l. Rectal examination
revealed no pelvic tenderness and sigmoidoscopy revealed a
normal rectal mucosa. Ultrasonic scan of the abdomen revealed
no evidence of gall stones. Later that day an exploratory
laparotomy was undertaken. At laparotomy no significant
pathology was detected. There was no peritoneal exudate. The
stomach, duodenum, gallbladder and liver all looked
macroscopically normal. The pancreas was slightly pink but
otherwise normal. The entire small bowel was inspected and no
abnormality was found. A solitary adhesion between the greater
omentum and the anterior abdominal wall was seen and
divided.

Questions:
 1. What other investigations would you have performed before
    proceeding to a laparotomy?
 2. What is your differential diagnosis?

Answers overleaf

2. 1. Blood, stool and urine cultures, extended Widal, liver function tests, urinary porphyrins.

2. Acute hepatitis, acute porphyria. The laparotomy findings really exclude such possibilities as enteric fever or brucellosis.

3. A 34 year old Nigerian Civil Servant was admitted with a two
week history of fever, headaches and malaise. For five days
prior to admission he had had a generalised maculo-papular
rash on the trunk and also upper and lower limbs including the
palms and soles. For three days he had had painful swelling of
the wrists and the knees and for two days he had had an
unproductive cough. P.M.H. Malaria as a child. Gastric ulcer 3
years previously, no recurrence. Social history: married with no
admitted extramarital relationships. Domiciled in England for
10 years.
On examination: febrile, temperature 39.5°C tachypnoeic,
tachycardia of 110/min. Small lymph glands both axillae.
Heart—no cardiac murmurs. Lungs—bilateral basal fine creps.
Abdomen—liver palpable 2 cms. below costal margin. Spleen
tipped. C.N.S. NAD. Skin-generalised maculopapular
erythematous rash. Joints tender, swollen left knee. Arthralgia
right knee and both wrists.

Investigations:

Hb 14.3 g/dl
WBC 6.6 × 10⁹/l (neutrophils 87%)
ESR 36 mm/hr
Plasma urea 4.4 mmol/l
    electrolytes normal
Serum bilirubin 7.5 μmol/l
    AST 135 iu/l
    alkaline phosphatase 131 iu/l
    total protein 50 g/l
    albumin 26 g/l
    calcium 2.26 mmol/l
    phosphate 1.28 mmol/l
HBsAg negative
Paul Bunnell negative
VDRL negative
Blood cultures; no growth

The swollen left knee was aspirated and clear yellow fluid
containing leucocytes, 60% of which were mononuclear cells,
was obtained. This was sterile on culture. No definitive
diagnosis was made. He continued to be pyrexial.

Questions:

1. What is your differential diagnosis?
2. What further investigations would you undertake at this stage?

Answers overleaf

3. 1. The differential diagnosis includes sarcoidosis, Hodgkin's disease, tuberculosis as well as a virus infection, possibly with an Echo virus.
2. Mantoux test, tomograms of the mediastinum, liver biopsy, axillary node biopsy and viral studies.

4. A 23 year old man was admitted complaining of sudden onset of generalised oedema. Ulcerative colitis diagnosed 9 years previously at the age of 14 when he had presented with diarrhoea and barium enema examination. Condition responded to treatment with Predsol retention enemas and Salazopyrin. Condition remained quiescent until three months prior to present admission when diarrhoea developed again and the patient lost 1 stone in weight. Steroid therapy had been recommenced in a dose of 10mg. b.d. which he was still taking at the time of admission.

On examination not anaemic, afebrile, blood pressure 160/100. Generalised swelling involving the face, abdominal ascites, scrotal oedema and bilateral oedema of the lower limbs.

Investigations:

Plasma urea 15.8 mmol/l
    creatinine 294 μmol/l
    sodium 136 mmol/l
    potassium 3.7 mmol/l
    chloride 106 mmol/l
    bicarbonate 17 mmol/l
Blood sugar 7.5 mmol/l
Serum bilirubin 13μmol/l
    AsT 20 iu/l
    alkaline phosphatase 131 iu/l
    total protein 41.7 g/l
    albumin 16.2 g/l
24 hour urinary protein excretion 4.5 G. Differential protein clearance 0.46.
IVP kidneys normal size, excretion of contrast material poor but not delayed.
Barium enema—ulcerative colitis involving rectum and descending colon.

Questions:

1. What would you consider to be the cause of this patient's fluid retention?
2. What further investigations would you perform?
3. The fluid retention responded to treatment. Subsequently, however, the patient complained of thirst and polyuria. What is the most likely cause for these new symptoms?

Answers overleaf

4. 1. The nephrotic syndrome. Although the urinary protein excretion was not as high as that usually found in the nephrotic syndrome this was probably due to the reduction in the level of the serum albumin at the time the urine protein was estimated. Whilst patients with ulcerative colitis may become hypoproteinaemic this is unlikely when the colitis is not extensive and in the absence of an associated anaemia due to blood loss.

2. Renal biopsy. This was carried out and electron microscopy showed evidence of widespread foot process fusion indicating minimal change nephrotic syndrome.

3. Hyperglycaemia and glycosuria induced by the combined effects of steroids and thiazide diuretics.

5. A 17 year old girl admitted complaining of headaches of six months duration mainly bitemporal and worse early in the mornings. There was nothing of note in her past medical history.
Drug history: Oral contraceptive prescribed 12 months previously but taken for only one month.
General examination was normal. Blood pressure 120/80. Examination of both optic fundi revealed papilloedema. Visual fields and visual acuity were normal and there were no other objective neurological signs.

Questions:
1. What is the most likely cause of the papilloedema?
2. What is the differential diagnosis?
3. What single investigation would you order?

6. A thirty six year old man was admitted following a grand mal convulsion. He had suffered from epilepsy since the age of two, with repeated grand mal episodes throughout his life resulting in five documented admissions for status epilepticus. His last admission had been two years beforehand, and on recovery it was noted that he had no abnormal neurological findings. He had been thoroughly investigated and the only abnormal investigation had been an electro-encephalogram.
In the two years since that admission, a progressive deterioration in intellectual performance had occurred with increased unsteadiness of gait. He had suffered an increased frequency of grand mal convulsions both during the day and at night, in spite of changes in his drug therapy. At the time of this admission he was taking phenytoin 550 mg daily and carbamazapine 300 mg three times daily.
After recovering from this present convulsion, he remained slightly sommolent. He had bilateral horizontal and vertical nystagmus with poor co-ordination of both arms and legs. He was unable to stand or walk without aid, with gross ataxia of his gait. He had normal power and tone in his limbs, with normal reflexes but bilateral extensor plantar responses.

Questions:
1. What is the most likely diagnosis?
2. What test would you do to confirm it?

Answers overleaf

5. 1. Raised intracranial pressure. The papilloedema is not due to optic neuritis because in this condition visual acuity is impaired. The blood pressure was noted to be normal and local causes such as venous occlusion can be excluded because the papilloedema was noted in both eyes.

2.(a) Pseudo-tumour cerebri
  (b) Obstructive hydrocephalus. Congenital or acquired. The absence of lateralising signs makes the presence of expanding lesions in the cranium such as neoplasm, abscess or subdural haematoma very unlikely.

3. Computerised axial tomagraphy of the head. This investigation will distinguish noninvasively between hydrocephalus in which the ventricular system is distended and a pseudo-tumour cerebri in which the ventricles are of normal calibre.

6. 1. Anticonvulsant intoxication.

Progressive cerebellar degeneration may be associated with long term phenytoin therapy.

2. Anticonvulsant levels in the blood.

7. A seventy year old woman was admitted following a sixteen hour history of continuous, lower abdominal, colicky pain. She had vomited, and passed several fluid motions during that morning. She had been unwell for the three previous days with a cough and green sputum and had complained of increasing thirst.

Her only previous admission had been following a right hemiparesis, from which she had made a good recovery. She was found to have mild hypertension and congestive cardiac failure, and because an embolus had been suspected, she had been given a course of anticoagulants. Thereafter she had been controlled on a thiazide diuretic alone.

On examination she was unkempt, drowsy and very dehydrated. The pulse was 90/min in atrial fibrillation, blood pressure 170/100 mmHg and temperature 35.6°C. In the chest, coarse crepitations were found at the right lung base. The abdomen was distended with vague tenderness and guarding in the right iliae fossa. Her bowel sounds were reduced and rectal examination revealed no abnormality. The CNS was normal.

Investigations:

Hb 13.9 g/dl
WBC 23.0 × 10^9/l (neutrophils 97%)
ESR 102 mm/hr
Blood glucose 37.6 mmo/l
Plasma sodium 152 mmol/l
       potassium 5.3 mmol/l
       chloride 119 mmol/l
       bicarbonate 21 mmol/l
       urea 25 mmol/l
Serum amylase 500 iu/l
Urine. Glucose 2%, ketones negative.

Two hours after admission the patient collapsed after passing a large melaena stool. Her pulse was 150/min and BP 80/60 mmHg.

Questions:

1. What condition has been precipitated by the right lower lobe pneumonia?
2. What is the most likely cause of her collapse after admission?
3. What immediate measures would you initiate?

Answers overleaf

7. 1. Hyperosmolar, non-ketotic diabetic coma.
2. Mesenteric infarction either due to an embolus, since she has had a previous embolic episode or a thrombosis due to the hyperosmolar state.
3.(a) Intravenous fluid replacement with potassium supplements.
  (b) Insulin infusion.
  (c) Parenteral broad spectrum antibiotic therapy.
  (d) Laparotomy.

Anticoagulants should not be given immediately after an embolic or thrombotic episode. They would predispose to haemorrhage within the infarcted region.

8. A thirty seven year old man was admitted drowsy, confused and disorientated in time and space. His wife had found him collapsed on the floor when she had returned home from work that same afternoon. He had been unwell for several days with increasing general malaise and night sweats. Over the previous twenty four hours he had become increasingly drowsy, and refused both food and drink, complaining that he felt nauseous. He had been started on prednisolone six weeks previously having been found to have pulmonary sarcoidosis, and he was taking 10 mg daily till the day of admission.

On examination, he had slight tachypnoea and mild dehydration. His temperature was 37.5°C, pulse 120/min. in sinus rhythm and blood pressure 100/60. The peripheral perfusion was reduced and he had central and peripheral cyanosis. The heart sounds were normal with no displacement of the apex beat. In his chest, he had dullness to percussion and decreased air entry with fine crepitations from the lung bases to mid zones. His abdomen was normal. In the central nervous system examination, he was found to have normal pupil responses and normal fundi. No neck stiffness was detected. He had poor movement of all limbs, with flaccid tone, normal reflexes and bilateral flexor plantar responses.

An initial chest X-ray showed bilateral hilar gland enlargement and confluent shadowing from both bases to the mid zones. On urine testing, a trace of protein and 1% glycosuria with ketones were detected.

Questions:

1. List three possible causes for the findings in this patient.

8. 1. (a) Bilateral bronchopneumonia with septicaemia and circulatory failure. This picture suggests an overwhelming infection possibly resulting from immune deficiency secondary to the corticosteriod therapy.

(b) Tuberculosis. There is no information on the evidence on which sarcoidosis was initially diagnosed.

(c) Acute adrenal insufficiency in a patient on steroids with an infection. This is unlikely after such a short time on low dose steroid therapy.

(d) Diabetic ketoacidosis.

9. An East African Asian aged 28 was brought to the Casualty department unconscious and was found to be severely hypoglycaemic. After treatment he was able to give a history. He had been treated for schistosomiasis three years previously but both before and since then had been suffering from bouts of dizziness, sweating and confusion, particularly if he had not eaten for a long time. He normally drank 4 pints of beer a day. On examination no abnormality was found. His BP was 110/70 mmHg with no postural fall.

Questions:

1. List the four most likely causes of his symptoms.
2. What is the significance of lack of postural fall in BP and the absence of abnormal pigmentation?
3. What four investigations would you consider in order to establish the diagnosis?

10. A man of 55 presents with unilateral exophthalmos and no symptoms or signs suggestive of dysthyroidism. There is a family history of hypothyroidism in his mother and Hashimoto's thyroiditis in his aunt.

Questions:

1. What three blood tests would be most useful in establishing a diagnosis of thyroid eye disease?
2. The tests are all normal. What further diagnosis would you consider?
3. What four further investigations would you do to make the diagnosis?

9.   1.(a) Cirrhosis of the liver due to schistosomiasis with alcohol induced hypoglycaemia.
     (b) Insulinoma.
     (c) Hypopituitarism (or solitary ACTH deficiency).
     (d) Addison's disease.
   2. They make the diagnosis of Addison's disease less likely.
   3.(a) Liver biopsy.
     (b) Fasting blood glucose with fasting plasma insulin.
     (c) Synacthen stimulation test.
     (d) Anterior pituitary function test (insulin, TRH & LHRH).

10.   1.(a) Total thyroxine may show hypo- or hyperthyroidism.
      (b) TRH test may show either a suppressed or an exaggerated response.
      (c) Positive thyroid antibodies would indicate an inherited pre-disposition to thyroid disease.
    2.(a) Tumour.
      (b) Infiltrative leukaemia or granuloma.
      (c) Cavernous sinus thrombosis.
      (d) Arteriovenous aneurysm.
      (e) Retrobulbar haemorrhage.
      (f) Orbital cellulitis.
      (g) Orbital periostitis.
    3.(a) Orbital CAT scan may show the thickened muscles characteristics of thyroid eye disease or the presence of a tumour.
      (b) Orbital ultrasound may show the enlarged muscles or a tumour.
      (c) X-rays of the orbit may show bony erosion due to a tumour or increased density of bone due to periostitis.
      (d) Angiography may show a vascular abnormality.

11. A man of 58 years was admitted to hospital complaining of malaise and weight loss over a few weeks. He was a heavy smoker and admitted to a productive cough for 20 years. There was also a history of shortness of breath on moderate exertion. Past history: usual childhood illnesses, fractured skull while playing rugby at age 25 years.
On examination: well developed man with evidence of some weight loss. Afebrile. Scattered coarse rhonchi throughout both lung fields. There was a grade 3/6 pan-systolic murmur at the apex radiating to the axilla. No other abnormal physical signs were found.

Investigations:
Hb 10.8 g/dl
WBC 9.8 × 10⁹/1 (Neutrophils 80%)
ESR 76 mm/hr

Chest X-ray showed increased lung markings and some old tuberculous changes at the right apex. There was slight enlargement of the heart.

Plasma sodium 128 mmol/l
potassium 4.1 mmol/l
chloride 96 mmol/l
bicarbonate 26 mmol/l
Liver function tests normal

Progress: he continued to lose weight and gradually became more breathless. Signs of congestive heart failure appeared with a raised JVP, enlarged liver and sacral oedema. The pansystolic murmur became louder and a pronounced 3rd heart sound appeared. A low grade fever also developed. Further investigation showed some deterioration in liver function with a slightly raised bilirubin and AsT. The ESR rose to 98mm in 1 hour. Blood cultures were negative.

Questions:
1. Suggest two investigations which might have helped in the diagnosis.
2. What was the diagnosis at post mortem?

Answers overleaf

11. 1.(a) Anti-streptolysin and anti-staphlolysin 0 titres.

The clinical course might suggest endocarditis although the patient was afebrile and blood cultures were negative.

(b) Sputum for malignant cells and possibly a bronchoscopy, particularly of the right apical bronchus for carcinoma which occurs in smokers and in old tuberculous scars.

2. Marantic endocarditis as a non-metastatic manifestation of carcinoma of the lung.

12. A white man of 28 years was admitted with a swollen, red and painful knee joint. He was noted to have a fever of 38°C. There were no other abnormal physical signs. Preliminary investigation revealed a white blood count of $18 \times 10^9/l$ with a neutrophilia.
The joint was aspirated of 100 ml. of yellow fluid containing neutrophils—this was sterile on culture.
The patient was given a broad spectrum antibiotic regime but the fever persisted. The joint stayed swollen and tender but both the fever and the swelling gradually improved despite stopping the antibiotic. Further investigations revealed an Anti-Streptolysin 0 titre of 156 units rising to 666 units subsequently. The HLA typing was B_{27} positive. Serum proteins showed a rise in alpha 2 globulins. An auto-antibody screen was negative. Rheumatoid latex test negative.

Questions:

1. Suggest two possible diagnoses.
2. What further tests would you do?

Answers overleaf

12.   1.(a) Rheumatic fever.
   (b) Ankylosing spondylitis.
   (c) Arthropathy associated with, but preceding inflammatory bowel disease such as ulcerative colitis or Crohn's disease.
   (d) Gout.
   2.(a) Serum urate level and examination of joint fluid specifically for urate crystals.
   (b) Investigations for inflammatory bowel disease are not indicated at this stage unless there is clinical evidence present.

13. A 65 year old woman developed resting tremor of the left hand and a diagnosis of Parkinson's disease was made. This was treated with benzhexol. Five years later she was bradykinetic and had generalised cogwheel rigidity which was more marked on the left side. She was started on L-dopa in doses increasing to 1250 mg/day over the next year and she improved markedly. When she was 75 her gait had deteriorated considerably and she tended to fall easily. She had occasional dystonic movements of the limbs. She was then on L-dopa 2g/day. At the age of 78 years she was admitted to hospital with confusion and urinary incontinence. She was unable to give a history but her daughter said that her tendency to fall had increased in the two years prior to admission. She had been housebound for 18 months. Three days before admission she had been found lying on her back on the floor and was unable to move. She had been incontinent of urine. Since then she had been confused and was unable to feed herself. Her incontinence of urine had recurred and she was once incontinent of faeces. Her mental state did not appear to fluctuate. Her drugs (L-dopa 500 mg q.d.s. orphenadrine 50 mg t.d.s. and diazepam 2 mg b.d.) had been administered regularly.

On examination she looked unwell. She was apyrexial. There was a pan-systolic murmur heard at the apex. There was a pulsatile swelling in the abdomen which was thought to be aortic in origin. She was disorientated in time and place and said very little spontaneously. There was no definite evidence of dysphasia. The cranial nerves were normal. There was marked axial rigidity, and cogwheel rigidity in all four limbs particularly on the left. She was very bradykinetic. She appeared to use the right limbs less than the left but power was probably normal on clinical testing. The reflexes were normal. The right plantar response was extensor. Sensation could not be adequately tested. She was just able to stand.

Haemoglobin was 12.5g/dl, white cell count 11.7 × 10⁹/l (68% polymorphs) with an ESR of 55 mm/hr. The blood urea was 10.5 mmol/l with normal electrolytes and liver function tests. Serum calcium was 2.61 mmol/l and phosphate 1.09 mmol/l. Blood glucose was 5.6 mmol/l. Urine culture was negative. Chest and skull X-rays and ECG were normal.

The day after admission the patient was slightly drowsy but was otherwise unchanged neurologically.

Questions:
1. What is the most likely diagnosis?
2. Which investigation would you perform urgently?

Answers overleaf

13. 1. The history of frequent falls in an elderly patient, followed by confusion accompanied by the suggestion of focal neurological signs, raises the possibility of a sub-dural haematoma. This may occur in the absence of headache, papilloedema or a fluctuating conscious level. The development of drowsiness makes a sub-dural haematoma the most likely diagnosis. At the time of admission the differential diagnosis included any of the causes of an organic confusional state. Chest or urinary tract infection were excluded. Both L-dopa and orphenadrine may cause confusion, this does not necessarily follow an increase in dosage. The patient could also have had a stroke involving the left cerebral hemisphere resulting in relatively minor neurological signs in the limbs.

2. A CT brain scan. This showed a low density left convexity sub-dural effusion which was compressing the left lateral ventricle and displacing the mid-line structures towards the right. A nuclear brain scan could also confirm the diagnosis but it is less reliable than a CT scan. Moreover, if a sub-dural haematoma is suspected, the patient should be transferred to a neurosurgical unit where CT facilities will be available.

14. A 56 year old woman went to the optician complaining of deteriorating eye-sight. She was immediately referred to an opthalmological clinic and found to have hypertensive retinopathy with perimacular exudates and flame-shaped haemorrhages. Her blood pressure was 250/140 mmHg and she had proteinuria.

She gave a history of attendance at a medical clinic for ulcerative colitis and spondylitis for 20 years. She had been controlled with oral corticosteroids until 10 years ago since when she had remained in remission without further treatment. Eight years ago she first complained of weakness of the legs and unsteadiness of gait. Six years ago during an admission for a lobar pneumonia she was found to have mild dysartharia, jerky bilateral nystagmus to lateral and upward gaze, marked incoordination of both arms and legs, ataxic gait, brisk tendon reflexes, bilateral ankle clonus with extensor plantar responses and impaired vibration sense in the legs. At that time her blood pressure was 140/85 mmHg. Her ESR was 115 mm/hr. LE cells were not demonstrated.

Chest X-ray and renal function studies were normal at that time. She was treated with oral corticosteroids for three months and had remained well in the next five years.

Questions:
1. What condition would you consider in the aetiology of her hypertension?
2. What one investigation would you do to confirm this?
3. What is the most likely cause of her neurological symptoms?
4. List two investigations which might be helpful in the diagnosis of this neurological disorder.

Answers overleaf

14. 1. Systematic lupus erythematosis. This might account for the lobar pneumonia, and high ESR.

2. Antinuclear antibodies particularly against double stranded DNA. LE cells are no longer used as a screening test for SLE since although they can ultimately be found in about 80% of patients the test may have to be repeated several times.

3. Multiple sclerosis.

4.(a) CSF for total protein and IgG
   (b) EEG for visual evoked potentials

15. A 17 year old boy was admitted in March 1981 complaining of pain of acute onset on the left side of the chest. Admitted to general ill health for a period of three months prior to this with anorexia, occasional fevers and a weight loss of more than 1 stone.
On examination thin and pale. Signs of left sided pneumothorax. Liver palpable 3 fingerbreadths below costal margin.

Investigations:

Chest X-ray—left pneumothorax
Hb 10.0 g/dl
ESR 80 mm/hr
Serum bilirubin 9.2 umol/l
    AsT 55 iu/l
    alkaline phosphatase >700 iu/l
    total protein 80 g/l
    albumin 34 g/l

Antinuclear antibodies negative. Antimitrochondrial antibodies negative. Ultrasonic scan—both lobes of the liver enlarged without evidence of biliary dilation.

Gall bladder and pancreas appeared normal.

A liver biopsy was performed but only a small sample of tissue was obtained. The liver tissue revealed an abnormal portal tract in which there was inflammatory changes suggestive of biliary tract disease. No definite diagnosis, however, could be made. His hospital course was complicated by the development of another pneumothorax on the right side which developed shortly after his liver biopsy. Eventually, however, his pneumothoraces resolved.

Questions:

1. Name six conditions that should be considered in differential diagnosis of his liver condition.
2. What further investigations would you perform? The patient was reluctant to undergo a further liver biopsy.
3. Subsequently the patient complained of diarrhoea and it was thought that there might be a connection between this and his liver disease. What would you now consider to be the most likely diagnosis?

Answers overleaf

15. 1. The six conditions that should be considered are chronic hepatitis, Hodgkin's disease or other reticulosis, sarcoidosis, hepatic tuberculosis, primary biliary cirrhosis and primary sclerosing cholangitis.

2. The investigations that should be performed are:
   (a) hepatitis B surface antigen
   (b) cholangiography, either by the percutaneous or retrograde route
   (c) barium enema examination together with sigmoidoscopy and rectal biopsy

3. The diagnosis is ulcerative colitis associated with primary sclerosing cholangitis.

16. A 53 year old woman was admitted as an emergency with left sided chest pain of sudden onset, pleuritic in type. P.M.H. bilateral cervical sympathectomies for Raynaud's disease. On examination afebrile, not anaemic or jaundiced. C.V.S. pulse 90/min, blood pressure 130/85 mmHg. No cardiac murmurs. No evidence of congestive cardiac failure. R.S. expansion diminished by pain but no localised pulmonary abnormalities. Abdomen—no masses palpable. Skin—bilateral cervical sympathectomy scars. Extensive brownish pigmentation with patchy areas of depigmentation. Several small telangiectases noticed on the hands.

Investigations:

Hb 12.8 g/dl
WBC 6.7 × 10⁹/l, normal differential

$WBC\ 6.7 \times 10^9/l$, normal differential

ESR 66 mm/hr
Chest X-ray normal
ECG—sinus rhythm. normal axis, no evidence of myocardial ischaemia or infarction or other pathology.
Lung scan—diminished perfusion and ventilation in the right upper lobe.
X-ray hands—O.A. changes right 1st carpometacarpal joint. Some calcification in the pulp of the 3rd phalanx at the tip.

Questions:

1. What further investigations would you perform to elucidate the cause of her chest pain?
2. The serum IgM level was found to be raised at 600 I.U. (normal 55-230). What other investigations would this finding lead you to perform and why?
3. The patient subsequently complained of dysphagia. What is the most likely explanation for this?

Answers overleaf

16. 1. Tests for antinuclear antibodies and other autoantibodies. Skin, muscle and lung biopsies might be considered as the high sedimentation rate suggests a collagen disorder.

2. Liver function tests and search for antimitrochondrial antibodies. A raised IgM level is seen in primary biliary cirrhosis, a condition which has been described in association with the C.R.S.T. syndrome i.e. calcinosis, Raynaud's phenomenon, sclerodactyly and telangectases. The patient exhibits the features of this syndrome, which may occur in isolation or as part of a generalised systematic sclerosis.

3. Oesophageal reflux with stricture formation secondary to oesophageal involvement from systematic sclerosis.

17. A lady of 58 years was referred to the Out-Patient clinic with a diagnosis of hypertension. On examination she was seen to have considerable vitiligo. The blood pressure was 190/115 mmHg. Heart normal. Chest clear. Abdomen—no masses or enlarged organs palpable. The fundi showed a little irregularity of arteriolar calibre. Testing of the urine albumin + with 24 hour excretion of protein 11.2g. WBC in urine 90/cu.mm.

Investigations:

Plasma urea	10.4 mmol/l
electrolytes	normal
Blood glucose	4.8 mmol/l
Haemoglobin	11.3 g/dl
Serum protein	62 g/l
albumin	29 g/l
paraproteins	8 g/l

Immunofixation showed kappa chains in the far gamma region.

Creatinine clearance 39 ml/min

Excretory urography and ultrasound showed a cyst in the right kidney. This was punctured and 16 ml. of yellow fluid obtained. Bone marrow aspiration and trephine showed no abnormality. A renal biopsy showed an end stage mesangiocapillary glomerulonephritis.

Progress. The creatinine clearance has not changed over two years. She remains anaemic and at present has considerable oedema. A trial of steroids in the past has not helped.

Questions:

1. List two further investigations which might be helpful.
2. How would you manage this problem?

Answers overleaf

17. 1. (a) Serum complement especially C_3 which is usually low in mesangiocapillary glomerulonephritis.

(b) Possibly repeat bone marrow or a radiosotopic bone scan to demonstrate areas of increased uptake to confirm a diagnosis of myelomatosis.

2. (a) Long term haemodialysis.

Renal transplantation is not indicated since mesangiocapillary glomeralonephritis tends to affect the transplanted kidney.

(b) Unless further evidence for myelomatosis were found no treatment is indicated at this stage.

18. A 26 year old woman 37 weeks pregnant was admitted to hospital in a state of diminished but fluctuating consciousness, having had no antenatal care. She had complained of headaches during the preceeding week. The baby was delivered vaginally, but one hour later she became deeply unconscious, with a pulse rate of 56/min, B.P. 70/40 mmHg with dilated pupils and neck stiffness and bilateral extensor plantar responses. The optic fundi showed no abnormality at that time.

The obstetrician thought she had meningitis, and a lumbar puncture was performed within four hours. The fluid was clear with a pressure of 290 mmHg., rising and falling on Queckenstedt's test. Analysis showed a WCC of 3 per cmm. protein 0.1 g/l. sugar 5.2 mmol/l and a gram stain showed no organisms.

Five hours later she had a period of apnoea and artificial ventilation was commenced. She subsequently developed a flaccid quadriplegia and died four weeks later without regaining consciousness.

Questions:

1. What three other diagnoses should have been considered initially?
2. What four investigations would you have performed to try and establish a definite diagnosis?
3. What was the cause of the deterioration following lumbar puncture?

Answers overleaf

18. 1.(a) Toxaemia of pregnancy, which would have been undetected in the absence of antenatal care.
(b) Subarachnoid haemorrhage.
(c) Cortical vein thrombosis associated with disseminated intravascular coagulation.
(d) Cerebral tumour.

2.(a) Repeated measurement of B.P.
(b) Urine for protein and red blood cells
(c) EMI scan if available
(d) Technetium brain scan
(e) EEG
(f) Carotid angiogram; R or L depending on development of appropriate focal neurological signs
(g) Prothrombin time, Fibrinogen level, Platelet count. FDP's

3. Coning of the cerebellar tonsils through the foramen magnum, resulting in cervico-medullary transection.

19. A 43 year old barman presented to his general practitioner with a four week history of pain in his thighs and calves, difficulty in climbing stairs and ankle swelling. He had lost one stone in weight over the last year, he drank five pints of beer and smoked 20 cigarettes daily.

On examination on admission to hospital one week later he was plethoric and generally thin. There was mild wasting of the shoulder girdle musculature and of the thigh muscles. There was mild proximal muscle weakness in the legs. The knee and ankle jerks were absent. There was bilateral ankle oedema, with tenderness of the calf muscles.

Investigations showed a normal haemaglobin with an ESR of 38 mm/hour and an MCV of 100. His asparate transaminase was 80 iu/l with an alkaline phosphatase of 110 iu/l and bilirubin of 18 μmol/l. Plasma CK was normal. Chest X-ray showed an opacity in the left lower lobe which was thought to be a carcinoma of the bronchus.

He was transferred to another hospital two weeks later. He said that the pain in his limbs had improved. On examination there was mild finger clubbing. There was slight weakness and wasting of the quadriceps femoris muscles bilaterally but no muscle tenderness or ankle oedema. The knee and ankle jerks were absent. There was subjective loss of pain appreciation below the knees.

Questions:

1. What is the most likely cause of the patient's neurological symptoms and signs?
2. Which investigation would confirm your diagnosis at the time of admission?
3. How would you treat him?

Answers overleaf

19. 1.   Alcoholic neuropathy. This may cause proximal muscle weakness which is often accompanied by pain, muscle tenderness and ankle oedema.Carcinomatous polymositis would be unlikely in view of the reflex loss in the lower limbs, the sensory loss, and the normal CK. A paraneoplastic polyneuropathy would usually present with more prominent sensory symptoms and signs and distal muscle weakness. However, the major diagnostic feature in favour of an alcoholic neuropathy is the fact that the patient improved after admission to hospital (with withdrawal of alcohol and improved diet). The suspicion of alcoholism raised by his occupation was confirmed by abnormal liver function tests and macrocytosis. His serum folate and vitamin B_{12} assays were normal. It is also unlikely clinically that his neuropathy was due to vitamin B_{12} deficiency. This produces prominent sensory symptoms with loss of vibration and joint position sense.

2.   Red cell transketolase estimation. This is a measure of thiamine deficiency.

3.   Parenteral administration of *B* vitamins, particularly thiamine, in high doses.

20. A 43 year old man attended Out-Patients in February 1981 with a history of swelling of both knees present for the whole of the previous 11 months, although the swellings varied in amount. His knees were stiff, especially the right, and particularly after work. They were sometimes, but not always painful. He had also noticed intermittent pain and occasional swelling of the wrists, and occasional stiffness of the fingers. There was no significant early morning stiffness. On direct questioning he stated that he had an occasional skin rash over the backs of his hands, and that his eyes sometimes appeared red and felt dry and irritant.

Past medical history. He had been admitted to hospital in 1979 with pericarditis of uncertain aetiology, which had subsequently cleared completely. At the time of his pericarditis he was found to have rheumatoid factor positive in high titre, but ANF was negative. His general health was otherwise good, and he had had no further time off work since he recovered from his pericarditis.

O.E. Healthy-looking man B.P. 120/70 mmHg, pulse 72 per min regular, heart sounds normal, lungs clear. Abdomen: liver edge palpable 3 cms below the right costal margin with a smooth edge. No other abnormalities. CNS normal. Skin clear. No lymphadenopathy. Locomotor system: there was a large effusion in the right knee and a smaller one in the left, but the knees were cool and movements full with slight discomfort on full flexion. There was slight swelling and tenderness of the right 2nd, and 3rd metacarpophalangeal joints, but at the time of examination all other peripheral joints and his spine were normal. 50 mls. of slightly turbid synovial fluid were aspirated from the right knee.

continued overleaf

20 continued

Investigations:

FBC Hb. 15.3 g/dl
WBC 9.4 × 10⁹/l
Platelets 167 × 10⁹/l
ESR 5 mm/hr.
Plasma urea & electrolytes normal
Serum total protein 80 g/l
  albumin 45 g/l
  globulin 35 g/l
  Protein electrophoresis: moderate to marked increase
    in gamma globulin
  calcium 2.65 mmol/l
  phosphate 0.86 mmol/l
  uric acid 0.42 mmol/l
  Rheumatoid factor (RAHA) titre l: 5120
  Antinuclear factor titre: l: 10

Questions:

1. What is the diagnosis?
2. Is this a common presentation of this disorder?
3. What investigations would you do ón the synovial fluid?
4. Mention one other investigation that you would order to confirm the diagnosis.

Answers overleaf

20. 1. Rheumatoid arthritis.

2. No. The most common presentation is a symmetrical polyarthritis (75%) affecting small joints of hands or feet (in 2/3) or large joints (approximately 1/3) or both in a few. 25% present with a monoarticular arthritis, most usually the knee. However, presumably this man's pericarditis was the first manifestation of his rheumatoid disease. While pericarditis occurs at some time in about 10% of those with RA, it is very unusual for it to be the presenting feature. In this respect his presentation is more like SLE. However, the fact that he has high titre rheumatoid factor and an ANF at first negative and then only 1 in 10 (insignificant) is more like RA, as were his X-rays which showed erosive changes in hands and feet.

3. Culture for gram positive and negative organisms and for tubercule. Examination for crystals, urate and pyrophosphate—note that he had a raised serum calcium and borderline high SUA.
Measurement of synovial fluid RF is not particularly helpful—it can be positive even in O.A., although a high titre might be significant.

4.(a) X-rays—especially chest, knees, hands and feet. Knees because clinically affected—hands and feet because the first characteristic X-ray changes of RA, especially the early erosions, usually appear there, and are likely to appear early in the feet whether clinically a problem or not. In this case there were already erosive changes in hands and feet.

  (b) Further auto antibody screen e.g. DNA binding.

21. A 41 year old man was admitted in May, 1981 with a two month history of increasing abdominal distension and dyspnoea on exertion. In July of 1980 after complaining of constant pain in the epigastrium and right hypochondrium for two months with anorexia and 12 lbs. loss in weight, he had been found to have a massively enlarged liver, 6cms below the costal margin. He admitted to an alcohol consumption of 4 bottles of spirits weekly for a number of years. Although liver functions tests were normal at that time a liver biopsy had shown areas of fibrosis present within the liver parenchyma in the region of the centrilobular veins. There were no other significant histological abnormalities and a tentative diagnosis of alcoholic liver disease with central hyaline sclerosis was made. In October of 1980 he had an episode of melaena for which no cause was found but in March of 1981 after further episodes of abdominal pain he was found on upper intestinal endoscopy to have a large duodenal ulcer. This was treated with cimetidine. His abdominal pain improved but he continued to be unwell.

On examination: not jaundiced, no lymphadenopathy. C.V.S. pulse 70/min regular, blood pressure 110/70 mmHg. Heart not enlarged, loud third heart sound./R.S. lungs clear/Abdomen—liver enlarged 4 cms. below the costal margin, and tender to palpitation. Abdomen distended with ascitic fluid.

Investigations:

Hb 14.3 g/dl
WBC 5.8 × 10⁹/l
ESR 8 mm/hr.
Blood urea 4.8 mmol/l
      electrolytes normal
Serum bilirubin 21.6 μmol/l
      AsT 31 iu/l
      alkaline phosphatase 131 iu/l
      total protein 72 g/l
      albumin 39 g/l

Questions:

1. What further investigations would you perform?
2. What diagnosis would you consider?

Answers overleaf
39

21. 1. Chest X-ray, ECG, measurement of central venous pressure, serum iron and total iron binding capacity, ascitic fluid tap, serum alphafetoprotein.

2. Constrictive pericarditis, constrictive cardiomyopathy, Budd-Chiari's syndrome, haemochromotosis with cardiomyopathy, hepatocellular carcinoma.

22. A 4 year old Jamaican girl was admitted as an emergency at 9.30 a.m. The child had woken up at 5 a.m. screaming and had a convulsion at 9 a.m. She had been reasonably well until the night before except for a cold and a cough of 3 days duration. She was known to have homozygous sickle cell disease. Had been regularly followed up in the clinic and had been taking regular folic acid medication. On admission she was unconscious, febrile (40°C) and pale with absent peripheral pulses. The blood pressure was barely recordable. Lungs clear and no focal neurological signs on clinical examination. Liver palpable 4 cm. and spleen not palpable.

Investigations:

Hb 7.0 g/dl
MCV 77fl
MCH 27 pg
Reticulocytes 8%
WBC 10.8 × 10^9/l (neutrophils 8.4, lymphocytes 2.4)
Platelets 54 × 10^9/l
Blood film showed target cells, Howell-Jolly bodies and an occasional sickle cell.
Urine and cerebrospinal fluid clear. No cells, no bacterial growth.
X-ray chest—lungs clear.
Blood glucose 5.8 mmol/l
Blood urea 6.2 mmol/l, electrolytes normal.
Coagulation screen—Prolonged thrombin time, 15 secs (control 12)
Fibrin degradation products present.

Progress: in spite of red cell and platelet transfusions, fresh frozen plasma and intravenous antibiotics, the child died within an hour of admission. Post mortem examination failed to show any evidence of bleeding.

Questions:

1. What was the nature of her terminal illness?
2. Could it have been prevented and if so by what measures?
3. Why was she prone to her terminal illness?

Answers overleaf

22. 1. Septicaemia, probably pneumoccal.
2. Yes (a) Antibiotic prophylaxis with penicillin
   (b) Pneumoccal vaccination
3. Hyposplenic state associated with sickle cell disease.

23. A fifty three year old woman presented with weight loss of five stones over a four week period. She complained of anorexia, tiredness and lack of energy during that time. She had suffered flatulence and repeated episodes of vomiting for a six week period, together with a change in her bowel habit. Her motions had become fluid, with a frequency of up to three times daily. The motions had previously been bulky and difficult to flush. Five years ago she had had a partial gastrectomy for a gastric ulcer which had not responded to medical treatment. Two years later, she had developed intermittent claudication of the right leg and had undergone a right aorto-iliac bypass graft. This had not been succesful and a mid-thigh amputation through the right thigh had been necessary.

On examination she was depressed, thin and wasted. She looked pale and had glossitis. Her hands and feet were warm. Her pulse was 120/min in atrial fibulation and blood pressure 160/80 mmHg. The cardiovascular and respiratory systems were otherwise normal, with no evidence of congestive cardiac failure. The abdomen was normal.

She was admitted for investigations. The results were as follows:

Haemoglobin 5.1 g/dl
WCC 1.4×10^9/l
Platelets 10×10^9/1
MCV 118 fl
MCH 32 pg
MCHC 35 g/dl
Film showed macrocytosis
Serum total protein 54 g/l
      albumin 33 g/l
A barium meal showed dilated small bowel with thickened mucosa and rapid transit time. A glucose tolerance test, xylose test, and jejunal biopsy were normal.

Questions:
1. What is the differential diagnosis?
2. What three further investigations would be helpful?

Answers overleaf

23. 1.(a) Vitamin B₁₂ deficiency following partial gastrectomy and consequent reduced intrinsic factor secretion.

(b) Post-gastrectomy steatorrhoea leading to fat malabsorption, folate deficiency and hypoproteinaemia.

(c) Carcinoma in the gastric remnant.

(d) Thyrotoxicosis is a remote possibility suggested by the recent rapid weight loss, diarrhoea, atrial fibrillation and hyperdynamic circulation.

(e) Malabsorption secondary to intestinal ischaemia is very unlikely inspite of premature atherosclerosis because of the lack of abdominal pain.

2.(a) Gastroscopy

(b) Barium meal

(c) Red cell folate which is superior to serum folate in assessing body stores

(d) Serum Vitamin B₁₂

(e) Possibly a Schilling Test

(f) Thyroid function tests

24. A 23 year old woman presented with a 5 week history of red
bumps appearing on the flexor surface of the hands, a rash on
the backs of the fingers, flushing of the face, and swelling and
stiffness of the fingers.

One week previously her legs had become swollen and she
developed pain in the feet, knees, hips and low back, and had
early morning stiffness lasting several hours. There was no
history of preceding infection.

She had a past history of a vagotomy for peptic ulcer 2 years
previously. On examination she appeared ill and had a
tachycardia of 110/min. She had a slight rash on the backs of
the knuckles and an obvious polyarthritis, with swelling,
tenderness and stiffness of the wrists, metacarpophalanges and
proximal interphalangeal joints of both hands. As she was
clearly ill she was admitted to hospital where she was treated
with bed rest and anti-inflammatory drugs. She did not improve
on this regime and after ten days in hospital her condition
deteriorated rapidly with the development of pyrexia up to
104°F, abdominal pain and vomiting, worsening of her arthritis
and the development of an extensive confluent, raised
erythematous rash spreading over the whole face, eyelids, arms,
upper trunk, and with shiny atrophic patches appearing in the
skin overlying the MCP and PIP joints and the patellae. The
skin was very tender to touch and she developed muscle
tenderness and weakness particularly in the shoulder girdles,
upper arms and thighs. She also developed crepitations at the
base of the right lung.

continued overleaf

24 continued

Investigations:

	7.3.80.	*18.3.80.*	*25.3.80.*
Hb.	12.3 g/dl	12.3	11.2
WBC	4.4 × 10⁹/l	6.8	8.6
Platelets	129 × 10⁹/l	189	330
ESR	46 mm/hr	59	95
AsT	114 units	138	47
CPK	160 units	165	165
γGT	70 units	74	63

Other investigations:

RA Latex	Negative
ANF	Negative
ASO titre	200 i.u.
Viral antibodies	Negative
Throat swabs	Negative
Sputum	Negative
MSU	Negative
Blood cultures	Negative
Australian Antigen	Negative
Monospot	Negative
Coomb's test	Negative

Total protein 83 g/dl
    albumin 39 g/dl
    globulin 44 g/dl
Urea & electrolytes normal
X-rays of chest hands and feet normal

Questions:
1. What is the diagnosis?
2. What two further investigations would you perform to confirm it?
3. What treatment would you give this patient?

Answers overleaf

24. 1. Dermatomyositis.

2.(a) Muscle & skin biopsy
 (b) E.M.G.

3. High dose steroids—60 mg/day in this case (and cimetidine in view of her history of D.U. and present abdominal pain and vomiting).

25. A 27 year old woman presented with an 18 month history of a rash appearing on and off over the face, and also involving the scalp, ears, foot and trunk at times. It was sometimes irritant and sometimes appeared following exposure to sunlight, but also at other times. Over the previous year she had developed tender finger tip lesions which healed with scarring of the finger pulps. Over the previous four months she had also noticed enlarged lymph glands in her neck and axillae, and over the previous 2 months she had developed occasional drooping of the eyelids especially when tired, which cleared spontaneously. She had been seen by another physician some four months previously who had found that she had a mild thrombocytopenia (platelet count 100—110 × 10⁹/1 on three occasions within a month) but she had never developed any petechiae.

On examination: pulse 76/min,   B.P. 140/70 mmHg

A faint maculopapular rash was present on the forehead and cheeks, right foot, left thigh, and abdomen. She had tender scarred lesions in the finger pulps of several fingers. She had multiple small, soft, but enlarged lymph glands in the neck, axillae and groins. Her spleen was just palpable. There was moderate thyroid enlargement, but no tremor or bruit. On that occasion the rest of the physical examination was normal.

Investigations:

Hb 11.9 g/dl
WBC 4.4 × 10⁹/l Normal differential
Platelets 88 × 10⁹/l
ESR 10mm/hr
Direct Coomb's Test negative
RA Latex test negative
ANF positive titre 1:160
VDRL negative
Viral antibody screen negative
Monospot test negative
Urine : protein +

Questions:

1. What is the most likely diagnosis?
2. Mention three further investigations you would wish to perform.
3. How would you explain the history of episodic ptosis in relation to your main diagnosis?
4. What further one investigation might you perform to elucidate this ptosis further?

Answers overleaf

25. 1. SLE

2. (a) Auto-antibody screen—especially for anti DNA antibodies or DNA binding. Other auto-antibodies e.g. ENA, RNP, SM.
   (b) Lymph node biopsy
   (c) Bone marrow examination
   (d) Complement levels.

3. The ptosis might be due to myasthenia gravis, which can be associated with other auto immune diseases— in this case with SLE.

4. Acetylcholine receptor antibodies.

Case Histories

26. A 70 year old woman was admitted with a ten week history of diarrhoea with blood in stools and tiredness and dizziness of same duration. She consulted her G.P. who started her on codeine phosphate 1g q.d.s. and Salazopyrin 0.5 mg. q.d.s. After two weeks she was referred to hospital as there was no response.
She was pale, not icteric and her lymph nodes, liver and spleen were not enlarged.

Investigations:

 Hb 8.2 g/dl
 MCV 73 fl.
 MCH 25 pg.
 WBC 5.4 × 10^9/l (normal differential count)
 Platelets 439 × 10^9/l.
 Reticulocytes less than 2%.
 Liver and reneal function profile normal.
 Sigmoidoscopy and biopsy showed ulcerative colitis.

Management was as follows:

 (a) 4 units red cells on admission, normalising the haemoglobin.
 (b) Prednisolone enema.
 (c) Prednisolone 40 mg. daily.
 (d) Salazopyrin 1.5g. q.d.s.

Progress: the diarrhoea progressively improved in the course of the next two weeks. Bleeding per rectum also ceased. However, after 3 weeks she was found to have a Hb. of 4 g/dl. MCV. 98 fl. MCH 32 pg. WBC 11.7 × 10/l, platelets 688 × 10^9/l, reticulocytes 8%. Direct antiglobulin test negative. Bone marrow aspirate showed adequate iron stores and normal iron in the normoblasts.

Questions:

 1. Name three possible causes of the anaemia at presentation.
 2. How should she be treated?

Answers overleaf
51

26. 1.(a) Salazopyrin-induced haemolysis
    (b) Autoimmune haemolytic anaemia which is associated with ulcerative colitis
    (c) Iron deficiency due to blood loss.
  2.(a) Discontinue Salazopyrin
    (b) Red cell transfusion

27. A man of 63 attended hospital complaining of swelling of the legs and breathlessness. He had smoked 20 cigarettes per day for most of his life. On examination he was cyanosed. There was a tracheostomy scar in the neck. (He said that this had been done some ten years previously following repair of a hernia). Jugular venous pressure was raised about 8 cm and there was gross oedema of both legs up to the thighs. The liver was enlarged four fingers breadths and was pulsatile. The right ventricular impulse on the precordium was prominent and there was a pansystolic murmur audible, maximal over the sternum. The $FEV_{1.0}$ was 1.4 litres, vital capacity 3.5 litres and peak expiratory flow rate just recordable at 70 l/min. Blood gases showed PCO_2 63 mmHg, PO_2 42 mmHg, pH 7.38.

Questions:
1. What was his cardiac murmur due to?
2. What two diagnoses would you consider as causative of his cardiac and respiratory failure?
3. What investigations would help to determine their relative contributions to his disability?

Answers overleaf

27. 1. Tricuspid incompetence
2. Chronic bronchitis, tracheal stenosis
3. Inspiratory and expiratory flow volume curves.

28. A 58 year old man attended the Out-Patient clinic in July, 1980 complaining of small haemoptyses over the preceding two months. He was a long-standing non-allergic asthmatic well controlled on prednisolone 5 mg/day and inhaled Salbutamol. He did not smoke and was otherwise well. There were no abnormalities on examination, apart from slight generalised wheezing, and peak flow was 385 l/min. Chest X-ray and ECG were reported as normal. Blood urea was 5.0 mmol/l, Hb 13.2 g/dl and ESR 17mm/hr

He was seen again in September, 1981 and reported that haemoptysis continued, with about one episode a month in which he coughed up small streaks of blood in his sputum for several days at a time. Chest X-ray was unchanged. Bronchoscopy was performed and no abnormality seen. He was followed up in the clinic. Haemoptysis continued. In May, 1981 he was admitted as an emergency following an anterior myocardial infarction with classical ECG findings and an LDH level of 1100 u/ml. He was treated with bed rest and anticoagulants.

Initial progress was good but after five days he had a sudden onset of chest pain on the right side with hypotension. The JVP was noted to be raised 6-8 cm and the liver enlarged 4 cm. Chest X-ray showed diffuse shadowing throughout both lung fields. Arterial PO_2 was 58 mmHg on 40% oxygen by mask, and PCO_2 27 mmHg. He recovered from this episode but the following week, suddenly collapsed. His pulse rate was 110/min, B.P. 70 systolic and his skin cold and clammy. There were no new ECG or chest X-ray changes. A few hours later he suffered a respiratory arrest, followed by an asystolic cardiac arrest from which he could not be resuscitated.

Questions:

1. What is the differential diagnosis of his haemoptyses?
2. What were the causes of his sudden episodes of deterioration while in hospital?
3. To what do you attribute his low PO_2?
4. What additional forms of treatment might have been given?

Answers overleaf

28. 1. (a) Recurrent pulmonary infarction
   (b) Idiopathic pulmonary haemosiderosis
   (c) Bronchiectases
2. Pulmonary emboli.
3. Ventilation/perfusion imbalance.
4. Streptokinase infusion or inferior vena cava ligation.

29. A 26 year old woman was found to have a systolic murmur at a routine medical examination. Subsequent investigation showed that she had aortic stenosis with a 25 mmHg gradient across her aortic valve. A year later she complained of pain and stiffness in her fingers in the morning and within a year had developed florid rheumatoid arthritis with a strongly positive Latex test. She was treated with non-steroidal anti-inflammatory agents, a course of penicillamine which had to be stopped because of oral ulceration, and then a course of sodium aurothialamate to a total dose of 750 mg. A month later she complained of breathlessness and chest X-ray showed both lung fields to be diffusely infiltrated with fine nodules. Lung function tests showed the following:

   Total lung capacity 3.3 litres
   Vital capacity 2.2 litres
   $FEV_{1.0}$ 2.0 litres
   T_LCO 6.3 ml/min/mmHg (Predicted 18.0)
   V_A (Alveolar Volume) 1.8 litres (Predicted 2.5)
   T_LCO/V_A 3.5 (Predicted >5)

Questions:

1. Describe what the lung function tests tell you in two short statements.
2. What is her residual volume?
3. What is the differential diagnosis of her lung problem?
4. What is the likely aetiology of her aortic stenosis?

Answers overleaf

29. 1. Small lung volumes with a "restrictive" ventilatory defect. Impaired gas transfer.
2. 1.1 litres.
3. Gold therapy, rheumatoid arthritis.
4. Congenital.

30. A man of 65 years was admitted with a history of sudden onset
of pain across the shoulders going around the chest. His legs
became very weak and he fell to the floor. At the same time he
became very short of breath. He had some paraesthesiae in the
legs and was unable to move them.
A week previously he had had a similar attack of pain lasting
for a few hours but this had not been associated with any
symptoms in the legs.

    P.H.   Right upper lobectomy for TB 8 years ago.
             Gastrectomy for D.U. 6 years ago.
             Bronchitis for many years.

On examination he was very cachetic. Blood pressure 70/30
rising to 140/80 mmHg. Peripheral pulses all present and equal.
Trachea deviated to right, some basal crepitations. There were
dilated veins on the abdomen which was soft. There was pain in
T5-6 region on neck flexion. Cranial nerves normal. There was
dense flaccid paraplegia with a sensory level at T5-6.

Investigations:

    Haemoglobin 10.6 g/dl
    WCC 11.0 × 10⁹/1—Normal differential
    ESR 9 mm/hr
    Electrolytes and blood urea—normal
    Acid phosphatase 1.3 K.A. units—normal
    Alkaline phosphatase 100 iu/l
    W.R. negative
    Plain X-ray of spine—normal
    Myelogram—no block
    CSF Protein 0.4 g/l—no increase in cells
    ECG ST segment raised and T inversion in anterior leads.

Anticoagulants were started but after two weeks he developed
melaena and these were stopped. Ten days later without any
improvement in his general condition or his parapalegia, he
contracted bronchopneumonia and died.

Questions:

    1. What was the diagnosis at post mortem?
    2. What investigations would you have done to make the
       diagnosis ante mortem?

Answers overleaf

30. 1. Dissecting aneurysm of the aorta leading to stripping of the small arteries to the spinal chord. This would explain the flaccid paralysis without any clearly demonstrable spinal chord lesion and would account for the very low initial blood pressure with the subsequent rise.

2.(a) Chest X-ray which might have shown widening of the mediastinum or a double aortic shadow

(b) Ultrasound or C.A.T. scan examination of the chest.

(c) An aortogram would be helpful in confirming the diagnosis but carries a risk.

DATA INTERPRETATIONS

1. A Negro woman who was found to have the sickle cell trait (AS) asked for her 15 year old son to be tested for the presence of HbS.

   His results were as follows:

Hb 10.5g/dl	Sickling test positive
RBC 5.06 × 10^{12}/l	HbS 70%
MCH 20.7 pg	Hb A 22.6%
MCV 64 fl	Hb A$_2$ 4.4% (N 2.5 to 3.7%)
MCHC 31.7%	Hb F 3%
	Serum ferritin 160 microgram/l

   Questions:
   1. What haemoglobinopathy does the boy have?
   2. What haemoglobinopathy would you expect to find on testing his father?

2. A 42 year old man being investigated for breathlessness is found to have the following results:

	Patient	Predicted
T$_L$CO	7.2	24.3 ml/min/mmHg
Alveolar Volume (V$_A$)	1.2	2.4 litres
T$_L$CO/V$_A$	6.0	Greater than 4

   Question:
   1. What do they reveal?

3. A 50 year old woman is admitted with a three-month history of generalised bone pains. Over the last month she has developed thirst, polyuria and constipation. Seven years previously she had a lump removed from her breast. Investigations showed:

   Serum calcium 3.2 mmol/l
          phosphate 1.7 mmol/l
          alkaline phosphatase 300 iu/l
          total protein 58 g/l
          albumin 32 g/l
   Plasma urea 9.5 mmol/l

   Questions:
   1. What are the two most likely diagnoses?
   2. What three investigations would you do to differentiate between them?

   Answers overleaf

1. 1. Sickle cell beta$^+$ thalassaemia.
2. Beta$^+$ thalassaemia.

The clinical and haematological manifestations of the double heterozygous state for HbS and beta-thalassaemia genes are very variable. Much of this variability is due to the two types of abnormal beta-chain synthesis. In beta$^+$ thalassaemia there is incomplete suppression and this is the usual type in Negroes and in parts of Italy. The complete absence of beta-chain synthesis in beta$°$ thalassaemia is found in Greece, S.E. Asia and Northern Italy.

2. 1. Impaired gas transfer due to loss of lung volume.

3. 1. Bone metastases from a carcinoma of the breast.
Primary hyperparathyroidism.

If the serum phosphate were low this would make primary hyperparathyroidism more likely, but since the blood urea is high, there may be phosphate retention associated with renal insufficiency so that the high phosphate does not exclude hyperparathyroidism.

2.(a) Bone X-rays to demonstrate secondaries or changes of hyperparathyroidism.

(b) Hydrocortisone suppression test. In about 70% of patients with hypercalcaemia due to malignancy the serum calcium will fall to a normal value within a week of hydrocortisone 150 mg daily, whereas in over 90% of patients with primary hyperparathyroidism it will remain elevated.

(c) Parathyroid hormone assay.

4. The following results were obtained in a 10 year old boy:
   Day 1, Midnight Plasma cortisol 83 nmol/l
      9.00 am Plasma cortisol 110 nmol/l
      9.02 am Synacthen 250 μg given intramuscularly
      9.30 am Plasma cortisol 110 nmol/l
   Days 1, 2, 3, Synacthen Depot 1 mg given intramuscularly at
      9.30 am.
   Day 4, 9.00 am Plasma cortisol 220 nmol/l
      9.02 am Synacthen 250 g given intramuscularly
      9.30 am Plasma cortisol 634 nmol/l

Questions:
   1. What is the diagnosis?
   2. What is the most likely cause?

5. A man with a venous haemoglobin of 16.7 g/dl smokes 30 cigarettes a day and has a carboxyhaemoglobin level of 10%. His P_{50} in vitro is 26.5 mmHg.

Question:
   1. What is the oxygen content of his blood at this PO_2? (Assume that 1g haemoglobin can bind 1.33 ml oxygen).

6. A 30 year old Irishman developed sore eyes and pains in his arms and legs.

Haemoglobin	14 g/dl
WBC	$5,600 \times 10^9/l$
ESR	75 mm/hr
Chest X-ray	Scattered mottling in both lung fields
Mantoux test	Negative
Serum calcium	2.8 mmol/l
phosphate	1.3 mmol/l
alkaline phosphatase	90 iu/l

Questions:
   1. What is the most likely diagnosis?
   2. Name three ocular lesions seen in this disorder.

Answers overleaf

4. 1. Hypopituitarism leading to adrenocortical insufficiency.

The normal response to Synacthen after three days of adrenocortical stimulation with Depot Synacthen shows that the initial failure of response was the result of adrenal atrophy due to lack of endogenous ACTH stimulation.

2. A pituitary tumour. In childhood this is most likely to be craniopharyngioma.

The same picture would be seen in a patient who had developed hypopituitarism as a result of prolonged steroid administration.

Other causes include primary or secondary malignant disease in the pituitary or hypothalamic region, infection such as tuberculosis or meningitis, granulomatous disease and trauma.

5. 1. 10 ml/dl.

10% of haemoglobulin is unavailable for oxygen carriage because it is carboxyhaemoglobin. Available haemoglobin is therefore 16.7 g/dl $\times$ 9/10 = 15 g/dl. Fully saturated this would carry 15 $\times$ 1.33 = 20 ml oxygen/dl. The P_{50} is the partial pressure at which the blood is half saturated, which is $\frac{20}{2}$ = 10 ml/dl.

6. 1. Sarcoidosis. Hypercalcaemia is found in up to 20% of patients.

2.(a) Lacrimal gland enlargement
   (b) Conjunctivitis
   (c) Keratitis
   (d) Iritis or uveitis
   (d) Cataracts

7. A 55 year old man has had similar liver function tests over
    several weeks.

    > Serum bilirubin $170\,\mu$mol/l
    >> aspartate transaminase 100 iu/l
    >> alkaline phosphate 400 iu/l

Questions:
1. What is the nature of his disorder of liver function?
2. Give three possible causes.

8. A 65 year old Londoner with bronchitis and airways obstruction
    has the following blood gas values breathing London air.

    > PO$_2$ 60 mmHg (8kPa)
    > PCO$_2$ 48 mmHg (6.4kPa)

    He wants to visit Denver, Colorado, altitude 5,000 feet (1600
    metres) atmospheric pressure approx. 630 mmHg.

Questions:
1. Would you advise him to go?
2. What precautions might he take?
3. Would you allow him to go to the Dead Sea?

9. A 60 year old man with a long history of excessive alcohol
    intake is brought into the Accident and Emergency department.
    He is drunk but complains of abdominal pain.

    > Plasma sodium 130 mmol/l
    >> potassium 3.5 mmol/l
    >> cholride 95 mmol/l
    >> bicarbonate 32 mmol/l
    >> urea 7 mmol/l
    > Blood glucose 5 mmol/l
    > Plasma osmolality 330 mmol/kg

Questions:
1. What is the calculated plasma osmolality?
2. Why does it differ from the measured osmolality in this
    patient?

Answers overleaf

7. 1. Cholestasis or obstructive jaundice.
2. Intrahepatic causes:
   Drugs such as chlorpromazine or methyltestosterone
   Primary biliary cirrhosis (but 90% are women)
   Ulcerative colitis
   Extrahepatic causes:
   Gall stone in the common bile duct
   Carcinoma of the common bile duct
   Carcinoma of the head of the pancreas
   Enlarged lymph glands in the portal fissure

8. 1. No—his arterial PO$_2$ would fall to about 30 mmHg.
2. He should use oxygen continuously.
3. Yes—his PO$_2$ would increase.

9. 1. 279 mmol/l.
Sodium concentration × 2 + potassium concentration × 2 +
glucose concentration + urea concentration all in mmol/l =
calculated osmolality in mmol/l.

2. Because alcohol is osmotically active and contributes to the
measured osmolality.

10. A Hindu woman of 35 who has lived in England for 6 years was investigated for increasing tiredness over the past few months. She had no loss of weight or gastro-intestinal symptoms and her periods were light. The following investigations were done:

Hb 9 g/dl	Serum B_{12} 50 ng/l
MCV 103 fl	Serum folates 15μg/l
RBC 2.8 × 10^{12}/l	Stools were negative for parasites
PCV 28%	and occult blood.
MCH 33 pg	Serum iron 5μmol/l
MCHC 31%	TIBC 86 μmol/l

Questions:

1. What is the likely cause of this woman's anaemia?
2. List two investigations that would confirm the diagnosis.

11. A 20 year girl is admitted unconscious to hospital:

Arterial blood pH 7.30	Blood glucose 4 mmol/l
PCO_2 3.5 kPa	Plasma urea 5 mmol/l
Bicarbonate 10 mmol/l	

Questions:

1. What is the likely cause?
2. What further test would you do urgently and how would this influence you management?

12. A 25 year old Cypriot man developed slight jaundice 5 days after appendicectomy. He had been given 2 pints of blood 24 hours earlier as his haemoglobin was found to be low, the FBC and film appearances having been normal on admission. He had also been treated for a urinary tract infection for the past 3 days with nitrofurantoin.

Hb 9.2 g/dl	Total bilirubin 55 μmol/l
MCV 89 fl	Conjugated bilirubin 10 μmol/l
MCH 31 pg	AST 36 iu/l
Reticulocytes 4%	Alkaline phosphatase 80 iu/l
Direct anti-globulin test	
negative	

Questions:

1. What is the probable cause of this patient's jaundice?
2. What test would you do to confirm it?

Answers overleaf

10.   1. Dietary deficiency of vitamin B_{12} and iron in a vegan.

2.(a) Marrow puncture to demonstrate both megaloblastic change and absence of stored iron.

(b) Reticulocyte and haemoglobin responses to small dose oral vitamin B_{12} and to iron therapy.

11.   1. Salicylate poisoning. The patient has a mild metabolic acidosis with a low PCO_2 and a low plasma bicarbonate. Other causes such as diabetic ketoacidosis or renal failure are excluded by the normal glucose and urea levels. Salicylates cause both a respiratory alkalosis by their stimulatory effect on the respiratory centre and a metabolic acidosis. As a result the pH may be relatively normal but there is a severe bicarbonate deficit.

2. Plasma salicylate. If the level is above 500 mg/l, forced alkaline diuresis should be initiated in someone with no evidence of renal impairment.

12.   1. Acute haemolytic episode precipitated by nitrofurantoin and infection in a patient with glucose-6-phosphate dehydrogenase deficiency.

2. G6PD screening test or assay of red cell G6PD activity.

The patient (and his doctors) should be advised on drugs to be avoided. In relation to urinary tract infections, sulphonamides and nalidixic acid may also cause haemolysis in patients with G6PD deficiency.

13. A 20 year old secretary complains of attacks of breathlessness on minimal exertion. During an attack of breathlessness in hospital she developed carpopedal spasm.

Serum calcium   2.5 mmol/l

		Predicted
FVC	3.5 l	3.81 l
FEV	3.0 l	2.91 l
P.E.F.R.	402 l/min	420 l/min

Questions:

1. What is the diagnosis?
2. How might an attack be terminated?

14. A woman of 55 years is admitted with a three day history of severe abdominal pain and vomiting. Twelve hours after an emergency operation for a perforated gastric ulcer she has passed no urine and urethral catheterization yields only 50 ml of urine. B.P. 90/60 mmHg.

Plasma urea	10.5 mmol/l
Urine sodium	10 mmol/l
Urine urea	140 mmol/l
Urine osmolality	650 mmol/kg

Questions:

1. What is the diagnosis?
2. What two lines of management would you institute?

15. A 35 year old man with a recurrence of peptic ulceration one year after gastric surgery.

Pentagastrin test

	Basal hour	0-15 mins.	15-30 mins.	30-45 mins.	45-60 mins.
Volume ml	80	25	20	25	15
pH	1.0	1.0	1.0	1.0	1.0
Acid mmol/ specimen	60	24	18	15	12

Questions:

1. What is the likely diagnosis?
2. What one biochemical test would confirm the diagnosis?

Answers overleaf
69

13. 1. Hyperventilation syndrome. This is a response to anxiety and young women are particularly susceptible. The lung function tests are normal.

2. Rebreathing from a paper bag.

14. 1. Renal circulatory insufficiency with uraemia.

The concentrated urine containing very little sodium indicates that the tubules are still functioning.

2.(a) Volume expansion with intravenous fluid.
  (b) Frusemide in high dosage.
  (c) The central venous pressure should ideally be monitored.

15. 1. The Zollinger Ellison syndrome.

The basal volume is high and the basal gastric acidity very high. Since the stomach is already maximally stimulated by endogenous gastrin there is no significant increase after Pentagastrin.

2. Fasting plasma gastrin assay.

16. A 16 year old Jamaican girl was admitted after an epileptiform seizure. She gave a six week history of abdominal pain. She subsequently developed a flitting arthralgia affecting wrists, elbows and shoulders. One week before admission to hospital she developed an effusion in the right knee joint.

Hb 10.3 g/dl	ESR 10 mm/l hr
WCC 4.2 × 10⁹/l	Rheumatoid factor negative
Neutrophils 19%	LE cell test negative
Monocytes 10%	Serum creatinine 110 μmol/l
Lymphocytes 70%	AsT 1000 iu/l
	Urine protein ++

Questions:
1. What is the most likely diagnosis?
2. What three tests would you do to confirm the diagnosis?

17. The following results were obtained in a man who had had a partial gastrectomy two days previously.

Plasma		Serum	
sodium 91 mmol/l		calcium 1.35 mmol/l	
potassium 2.8 mmol/l		phosphate 0.3 mmol/l	
chloride 67 mmol/l		total proteins 45 g/l	
bicarbonate 12 mmol/l			
urea 3.9 mmol/l			

Questions:
1. What is the likely cause?
2. What investigation would you do next?

18. The following results were obtained from a cardiac catheter in a 53 year old man who was being investigated for a systolic murmur after a myocardial infarct.

Pressures mmHg	Oxygen saturation %
RA 8 mean	74%
PA 50/18	84%
PAW 18 mean	
LV 95/18	94%
AO 95/60	94%

Questions:
1. What is the diagnosis?
2. What would be ideal management if patient remains stable?

Answers overleaf

16. 1. Systemic lupus erythematosis.

Rheumatoid arthritis or rheumatic fever are less likely.

2. (a) Anti-double stranded DNA antibody-present in 99%
    (b) Chest X-ray
    (c) EEG
    (d) Brain scan
    (e) Lumbar puncture

The LE cell test is positive in 80% of unequivocal cases but it may be necessary to repeat it several times and it has been superseded by (a).

17. 1. The blood had been obtained from a venepuncture done in the arm into which a dextrose drip was running. The "blood" is diluted with dextrose giving these low results.

2. Repeat the tests on blood taken from the other arm.

18. 1. Post-infarct ventricular septal defect.

2. Maintain for at least six weeks after the infarct before undertaking surgical correction.

19. A 70 year old man was admitted with chest pain. Enzyme results on admission:

		Normal range
Serum creatine kinase	180 iu/l	10-100 iu/l
aspartate transaminase	30 iu/l	5-40 iu/l
alphahydroxybutyrate dehydrogenase	120 iu/l	50-150 iu/l

Question:
1. What event do these results indicate and when?

20. Six days later the following results are obtained in the same patient.

Serum creatine kinase	440 iu/l
aspartate transaminase	120 iu/l
alphahydroxybutyrate dehydrogenase	310 iu/l

Question:
1. What is the cause of these results?

21. CSF from a 6 year old girl was turbid and contained 2,560 × 10^6 WBC/l. Large numbers of gram-negative diplococci were seen.

Questions:
1. What is the most likely organism?
2. What is the appropriate antibiotic?

22. A 27 year old girl is seen in the Accident and Emergency Department with a history of having taken 30 paracetamol tablets two hours previously.

Plasma paracetamol 400 mg/l
Serum aspartate transaminase 25 iu/l

Question:
1. What two lines of therapy would you initiate?

Answers overleaf

19. 1. A myocardial infarct 4-6 hours before the blood sample was taken.

The creatine kinase starts to rise about 4 hours after an infarct and the aspartate transaminase about 6 hours after an infarct.

20. 1. Reinfarction.

The creatine kinase and aspartate transaminase levels would have returned to normal six days after the first infarct if there had been no further myocardial damage.
The raised alphahydroxybutyrate dehydrogenase is still due to the first infarct since levels of this enzyme remain elevated for 7-10 days.

21. 1. Neisseria meningitides.
　　　 2. Benzyl penicillin.

22. 1.(a) Gastric aspiration and lavage should be undertaken if the patient is admitted within 4 hours of taking the tablets.

　(b) N-acetylcysteine is indicated in someone whose plasma paracetamol level is above a line (on semi-logarithmic paper) joining 200 mg/l at 4 hours to 30 mg/l at 15 hours. Treatment should not await the results of investigations if the patient has taken more than 7.5g or the overdose was taken 8-15 hours before admission. If the plasma is later found to be below the treatment line, the treament can be stopped.

After 15 hours it is too late for treatment to be effective and it may harm patients once they have developed liver damage.

23. A 43 year old man is found to have glycosuria at an Insurance medical examination.

A glucose tolerance test gives the following results:

	Fasting	½hr	1hr	1½hr	2hr
Blood glucose (mmol/l)	5.0	11.5	7.5	2.5	4.0
Urine glucose	Negative		Negative		Negative

Question:

1. What event in his past medical history might account for these results?

24. A 27 year old woman ruptured her uterus during delivery at term of her 4th child. She had severe uterine haemorrhage and hypotension and underwent an emergency hysterectomy. During the next year she complained of weight loss and polyuria. Blood glucose, plasma electrolytes, serum calcium and serum total T4 were all normal. Her urine output was 6.5 1/24 hrs.

A combined anterior pituitary stimulation with insulin TRH and LHRH gave the following results:

Time minutes	Glucose mmol/l	Cortisol nmol/l	GH mU/l	TSH mU/l	LH U/l	FSH U/l
0	5.0	290	5	3	3.6	2.3
30	2.0	450	25	10	10.9	6.5
60	2.3	700	22	8	40	10.2
90	3.2	500	12			
120	4.5	500	8			

Questions:

1. What possible diagnosis would you consider?
2. What one biochemical investigation would you do next to establish the diagnosis?

25. A 30 year old asymptomatic woman whose older brother had recently died suddenly, has a 4/6 systolic ejection murmur heard best between the apex and the left sternal edge which decreases in intensity when she is in the squatting position, a fourth heart sound and a jerky carotid pulse. ECG shows Q waves in the inferior leads and widespread ST-T changes.

Questions:

1. What is the diagnosis?
2. What two findings might you expect on echocardiography in this patient?

Answers overleaf

23. 1. Gastrectomy or gastroenterostomy.

This is a lag storage curve. It is also seen in normal patients with no medical disorder, in severe liver disease and hyperthyroidism.

24. 1. Diabetes insipidus.

This is a very rare complication of intra-partum haemorrhage. It is more usual for the anterior pituitary to suffer than the posterior pituitary but in this case the anterior pituitary response to stimulation is entirely normal.

2. A vasopression test with DDAVP (1 – desamino 8 – arginine vasopression) intranasally or intramuscularly should lead to a fall in the urine flow rate and a steep rise in the urine osmolality within 2 hours.

25. 1. Hypertrophic cardiomyopathy.
2.(a) Asymmetrical septal hypertrophy.
  (b) Systolic anterior movement of mitral valves.
  (c) Early closure of aortic valve.

26. A 53 year old man, a known diabetic on sulphonylurea tablets presents with profuse glycosuria and ketonuria.

Blood glucose   27 mmol/l
Arterial blood   pH 7.10
                    PCO2 8.2 kPa
                    bicarbonate 17 mmol/l

Questions:
1. What type of hydrogen ion disturbance do these results indicate?
2. What is the most likely cause?

27. A 30 year old woman presents with anorexia, nausea and tiredness for several weeks and itching for 5 days. She is jaundiced with palpable liver and spleen. She has not taken any drugs.

Serum bilirubin   180 μmol/l
    asparate transaminase   750 iu/l
    alkaline phosphatase   150 iu/l
    total protein   67 g/l
    albumin   23 g/l

Questions:
1. What two diagnoses would you consider?
2. Name three investigations which might help to differentiate between them.

28. A premature neonate has the following blood gas results:

	10 p.m.	6 a.m.
Arterial pH	6.95	7.58
PCO$_2$	8.5	3.1 kPa
bicarbonate	12	25 mmol/l
PO$_2$	3.8	22.3 kPa

Question:
1. What is the likely cause of the final metabolic disturbance?
2. Name a potential complication of this situation.

Answers overleaf

26. 1. Combined metabolic and respiratory acidosis. The low pH is the result of both carbon dioxide retention and bicarbonate depletion.

2. A chest infection producing a worsening of the diabetes and impaired respiratory compensation of the metabolic ketoacidosis.

27. 1.(a) Infective hepatitis.
    (b) Chronic active hepatitis.

The very high transaminase and slightly raised alkaline phosphatase indicate hepatocellular damage. The low albumin suggests that the damage is extensive and prolonged. This degree of hypoalbuminaemia is not usually seen in infective hepatitis.

2.(a) Hepatitis Bs antigen. This can be detected in infective hepatitis before the onset of symptoms and for several weeks afterwards. It is not found in 90% of patients with chronic active hepatitis.

    (b) Anti-nuclear factor present in about half the patients with CAH.

    (c) Smooth muscle antibody present in two thirds of patients with CAH.

    (d) Liver biopsy.

28. 1. Overventilation with oxygen resulting in a respiratory alkalosis in a baby with the respiratory distress syndrome.

2. Retrolental fibroplasia resulting from excessive oxygen therapy.

29. A 53 year old woman with a history of excessive bruising which she first noticed five years previously after a minor fall is obese and her blood pressure is 200/100 mmHg.

Plasma sodium	142 mmol/l
potassium	3.3 mmol/l
chloride	96 mmol/l
bicarbonate	31 mmol/l
urea	6 mmol/l
Serum total protein	72 g/l
Random blood glucose	12 mmol/l
Platelets	$200 \times 10^9/l$
Bleeding time	7 minutes

Prothrombin time, partial thromboplastin time, thrombin clotting time, all normal.

Questions:

1. What is the most likely diagnosis?
2. What three biochemical investigations would you do to confirm it?

30. A 40 year old woman complaining of urinary frequency and occasional swollen ankles.

24 hour urine volume 2880ml
Urine creatinine 4.4 mmol/l = $4400\,\mu$mol/l
Serum creatinine 88 μmol/l
Creatinine clearance 10 ml/minute

Question:

1. What is the reason for this creatinine clearance result?

31. A 35 year old man is found to have glycosuria at an Insurance medical examination.

A glucose tolerance test gives the following results:

	Fasting	½hr	1hr	1½hr	2hr
Blood glucose (mmol/l)	4.1	6.1	7.7	6.6	4.4
Urine glucose	Negative	Positive +		Positive ++	

Questions:

1. What is the diagnosis?
2. What treatment is indicated?

Answers overleaf

29. 1. Cushing's syndrome. The combination of hypertension, hypokalaemic alkalosis and hyperglycaemia is characteristic of glucocorticosteroid excess.

2 (a) Plasma costisol levels at 9 a.m. and midnight.
  (b) Plasma ACTH levels at 9 a.m. and midnight.
  (c) Dexamethasone suppression test.

These three tests should confirm Cushing's syndrome and give a good indication of the aetiology.

30. 1. The calculation is incorrect.
The formula for the clearance calculation is:

$$\frac{\text{Urine concentration } (\mu\text{mol/l})}{\text{Serum concentration } (\mu\text{mol/l})} \times \frac{\text{24hr urine vol. (ml)}}{1440} \text{ ml/minute}$$

1440 is the number of minutes in 24 hours.

The correct answer is therefore

$$\frac{4400}{88} \times \frac{2880}{1440} = 100 \text{ ml/minute}$$

Since the serum creatinine is normal and the urine volume is high it is most unlikely that the clearance would be reduced.

31. 1. Renal glycosuria.
  2. None.

32. Investigations in a 50 year old man with oedema and ascites gave the following results:

    Serum total protein 45 g/l
           albumin 18 g/l
           cholesterol 12.3 mmol/l
           total thyroxine 45 nmol/l
           TSH 5 mU/l

Urine showed heavy proteinuria and moderate glycosuria.

Questions:

  1. What is the diagnosis?
  2. Name three possible underlying causes.
  3. What is the significance of the thyroid function tests?

33. A 10 year old boy with acute lymphoblastic leukaemia has been treated with vincristine and prednisolone.

  Hb 12.5 g/dl   Normal differential with no abnormal cells
  WBC $5.3 \times 10^9/1$ Platelets $220 \times 10^9/1$

Bone marrow shows regeneration and is free from leukaemia blast cells.

Question:

  1. What further treatment would you give?

34. A 50 year old man complained of pruritus.

Hb 21.5 g/l	MCHC 30 g/dl
Red cell count 8×10^9/dl	Serum bilirubin 18 μmol/l
PCV 0.65	Uric acid 0.52 mmol/l
MCV 81 fl	Blood glucose 5 mmol/l
MCH 27 pg	

Questions:

  1. What is the diagnosis?
  2. What three tests would you do to confirm the diagnosis?

35. Sputum from a 60 year old man with a severe acute exacerbation of chronic bronchitis yields Haemophilus influenzae, coliforms and Streptococus viridans.

Questions:

  1. Which is the most likely pathogen?
  2. What is the antibiotic of choice?

Answers overleaf

32. 1. Nephrotic syndrome, in which increased glomerular permeability leads to proteinuria (by definition more than 5g daily) and therefore hypoalbuminaemia and oedema. There is also hyperlipoproteinaemia.

2.(a) Diabetes mellitus, which is likely in this case because of the glycosuria.
  (b) Glomerulonephritis (about 80% of nephrotics)
  (c) Systemic lupus erythematosis.
  (d) Renal amyloidosis.
  (e) Inferior vena cava or renal vein thrombosis.

3. The low thyroxine is due to a low level of thyroid binding protein which is also characteristic of the nephrotic syndrome. The normal TSH shows that the patient is not hypothyroid.

33. 1.(a) Prophylactic skull irradiation and intrathecal methotrexate. This should be given to all children with acute lymphoblastic leukaemia once remission has been induced. Over half the patients develop CNS leukaemia after successful haematological remission unless they are given prophylaxis.

  (b) Maintenance cytotoxic therapy for at least 120 weeks. There are various protocols using combinations of mercaptopurine, methotrexate,vincristine and prednisolone or other drugs.

34. 1. Polycythaemia rubra vera.
Pruritus occurs in two-thirds of patients although it is rarely the presenting symptom. It does not occur in secondary polycythaemia.

2.(a) White cell and platelet counts.
These are high in three-quarters of patients with PRV.
  (b) Red cell volume and plasma volume.
  (c) Arterial oxygen saturation.
  (d) Leukocyte alkaline phosphatase.

35. 1. Haemophilus influenzae.
2.(a) Ampicillin or amoxycillin orally, or parenterally if the patient is very unwell.
  (b) Chloramphenicol which diffuses rapidly into respiratory secretions. Resistance is rare and toxicity is most unlikely if it is given only for 5 days.

36. A 50 year old man, a heavy cigarette smoker with a long history of chronic bronchitis has lost two stones in weight over the past year. Over the past six weeks he has become increasingly weak.

Plasma sodium	115 mmol/l
potassium	6.5 mmol/l
chloride	80 mmol/l
bicarbonate	13 mmol/l
urea	29 mmol/l

Questions:

1. What is the likely diagnosis?
2. What one test will support or refute the diagnosis?

37. A one year old girl admitted for investigation of failure to thrive and hepatomegaly. After fasting the following results were obtained:

	12 hours	*18 hours*
Blood glucose	2.1 mmol/l	0.5 mmol/l
lactate	3.5 mmol/l	8.5 mmol/l (Normal 1-2 mmol/l)
pH	7.40	7.17

Questions:

1. What is the most likely diagnosis?
2. What investigation will confirm this diagnosis?

38. A 60 year old man has a long history of ventilatory insufficiency due to old pulmonary tuberculosis. He is admitted to hospital with increasing dyspnoea, cyanosis and pyrexia.

On admission:

Arterial pH 7.43
PCO_2 8.7 kPa (64 mm Hg)
bicarbonate 42 mmol/l

Question:

1. What acid base disturbance does he have?

Answers overleaf

36. 1. Addison's disease, either autoimmune or tuberculous or metastatic destruction of the adrenals.

2. Failure of plasma cortisol to rise after Synacthen.

37. 1. Glycogen storage disease Type 1 (Von Gierke's disease) is is due to glucose-6-phosphatase deficiency and there is fasting hypoglycaemia with lactic acidosis.

2. Liver biopsy with assay of hepatic glucose-6-phosphatase activity.

38. 1. Compensated respiratory acidosis.

The pH is normal in spite of considerable carbon dioxide retention. In patients with chronic respiratory insufficiency buffer base is retained to compensate for the carbon dioxide retention and there may be no fall in the arterial blood pH with a PCO_2 of up to 10 kPa.

39. After 4 hours of assisted ventilation his blood gas results are found to be

Arterial pH 7.57
  PCO_2 5.3 kPa (40 mm Hg)
  bicarbonate 36 mmol/l

Question:

1. What acid base disturbance does he now have?

40. A woman of 32 is admitted for investigation of abdominal pain:

Plasma sodium	141 mmol/l
potassium	7.8 mmol/l
chloride	102 mmol/l
bicarbonate	24 mmol/l
urea	4.5 mmol/l
Blood glucose	4.0 mmol/l

Question

1. What is the most likely cause of these results?

41. A man of average height, 60 years old, has the following values on lung function testing:

$FEV_{1.0}$ 1.2 litres (40% Predicted Normal)
Vital Capacity 3.1 litres (75% Predicted Normal)
Static pulmonary compliance 0.64 l/cmH$_2$0 (Normal 0.2-0.5)

There was no change after bronchodilator aerosol.

Questions:

1. What are his physiological abnormalities?
2. What are the likely pathological changes in his lungs?

39. 1. Metabolic alkalosis.

Ventilation has reduced his carbon dioxide level to normal but increased renal excretion of the previously raised bicarbonate has not kept pace.

40. 1. Haemolysis of the red blood cells or delay in transport of the blood to the laboratory leading to leakage of potassium from the red cells into the plasma before there is visible haemolysis.
In view of the normal bicarbonate, urea and glucose hyperkalaemia is not due either to a renal cause or to diabetic ketoacidosis.

41. 1. Irreversible airways obstruction and hypo-elastic lungs.
2. Panacinar emphysema.

42. A 7 year old boy reached his chief milestones late. His mother says he always seems tired, and suffers from constipation. Two years previously his scalp hair had become thin and his fingernails flaky. Recently he has complained of tingling in his fingers and cramps in his legs.

Hb 12.7 g/dl
Serum calcium 1.5 mmol/l
       phosphate 3.2 mmol/l
       alkaline phosphatase 290 iu/1
Production of transfer factor to candida antigen
   50% of normal for his age.

Questions:
1. Name two likely diagnoses?
2. What three further investigations should be performed?

43. Urine from a 26 year old women in the third trimester of pregnancy who has symptoms of a urinary tract infection shows a significant growth of Esch.Coli sensitive to ampicillin, tetracycline and co-trimoxazole.

Questions:
1. Which antibiotic should you prescribe?
2. What are the contra-indications to the other two?

44. A 55 year old man had the following blood count:

Hb	19 g/dl
PCV	0.54
RBC	$6.5 \times 10^9/1$
MCV	84 fl
MCHC	35 g/dl
MCH	29 pg
WBC	$8.5 \times 10^9/1$
Platelets	$200 \times 10^9/1$
Arterial PO_2	11.0 kPa
Red cell volume	normal
Plasma volume	slightly reduced

Questions:
1. What is the diagnosis?
2. What treatment is indicated?

Answers overleaf

42. 1.(a) Idiopathic hypoparathyroidism
(b) Pseudohypoparathyroidism

2.(a) Parathyroid hormone assay

In hypoparathyroidism there is deficiency of the hormone, whereas in pseudohypoparathyroidism there is failure of receptor response to the hormone which is secreted normally.

(b) Urinary cyclic AMP after PTH infusion. This will rise in hypoparathyroidism but in pseudohypoparathyroidism there is no response.

(c) Bone X-rays for increased density and short metacarpals, metatarsals and phalanges.

43. 1. Ampicillin.

2. Tetracycline binds to calcium ions in bones and tooth buds. It may cause discoloration of teeth and there is also a remote possibility of retardation of bone and tooth growth in the foetus.

Co-trimoxazole is an inhibitor of folate metabolism and might exacerbate folate depletion in pregnancy.

44. 1. Pseudopolycythaemia or polycythaemia of stress.

The normal white cell and platelet counts rule out polycythaemia rubra vera, the normal PO_2 hypoxic secondary polycythaemia and the normal red cell volume, secondary polycythaemia without hypoxia.

2. None. The marrow is not hyperplastic so that P^{32} treatment is contra-indicated.

45. The following results are obtained from a six week old baby
whose mother says he is constantly thirsty and is passing large
quantities of urine:

Plasma sodium	144 mmol/l
potassium	4 mmol/1
chloride	106 mmol/l
bicarbonate	28 mmol/l
Plasma osmolality	305 mmol/kg
Urine osmolality	120 mmol/kg

After intra-nasal DDAVP (1 – desamino – 8 – D arginine
vasopressin) his urine osmolality fails to rise.

Questions:

1. What is the diagnosis?
2. What investigation would confirm the diagnosis?

46. A 16 year old girl at an employment medical examination is
found to have a palpable firm spleen. She has had two attacks
of mild jaundice over the last year with no other symptoms.
Her father also had jaundice until he had an operation. She is
not on any drugs.

Hb 11.0 g/dl	MCH 29 pg
MCV 89 fl	MCHC 37 g/dl, Reticulocytes 5%

On a film red cells were reported to be spherocytic.

Serum bilirubin 25 μmol/l
Urine: no bile, urobilinogen present

Questions:

1. What is the likely diagnosis?
2. What treatment would you advise?

47. A 19 year old unmarried girl with a history of Graves' disease
for which carbimazole was prescribed, is seen in the ante-natal
clinic where pregnancy is confirmed. Her pulse rate is
136/minute.

Serum total thyroxine 300 nmol/l
Thyroid hormone uptake test 94% (normal 93-117%)
Free thyroxine index 32 (normal 5.5-16)
Serum free thyroxine 28 pmol/l (normal 9-22 pmol/l)

Questions:

1. What do these results indicate?
2. What is the most likely cause?

Answers overleaf

45. 1. Nephrogenic diabetes insipidus.

2. Plasma vasopressin although this is only necessary if osmolality studies are equivocal. In nephrogenic diabetes insipidus it will be high where as in pituitary diabetes insipidus it will be low.

46. 1. Hereditary spherocytosis.
Spherocytosis may be congenital or acquired as the result of auto-immune haemolytic anaemia, chemicals, infections or burns. In this case there is a very suggestive family history and no evidence of any other cause.

2. Splenectomy, since even if the haemolysis is well compensated, more than half the patients will develop gall-stones.

47. 1. Persistent thyrotoxicosis. The total thyroxine, free thyroxine and free thyroxine index are all raised. The thyroid hormone uptake test is within the normal range because of the increase in thyroid binding protein in pregnancy which has the opposite effect on the test from that of hyperthyroidism.

2. Failure of the patient to take her medication.

48. The importance of taking her tablets is emphasised to the above girl. A month later she is seen again and now appears mildly hypothyroid.

> Serum total thyroxine, less than 20 nmol/l
> Thyroid hormone uptake test 125% (normal 93-117%)
> Free thyroxine index, less than 2 (normal 5.5-16)
> TSH 5 mu/l (normal up to 10 mu/l)

Questions:

1. What do these results indicate?
2. Why is the TSH normal?

49. A 35 year old man is found to have a blood pressure of 180/110mm Hg. He is started on a thiazide diuretic. After one month's treatment the following biochemical results are obtained:

Plasma sodium	145 mmol/l
potassium	2.2mmol/l
chloride	102 mmol/l
bicarbonate	31 mmol/l
urea	7.5 mmol/l
Plasma cortisol 9 a.m.	500 mmol/l
12 midnight	240 mmol/l

Questions:

1. Name three conditions which you would consider in the differential diagnosis
2. What three tests would you do to differentiate between them?

50. A 40 year old housewife with a history of increasing dyspnoea has central cyanosis, finger clubbing and fire rales at both bases.

Chest X-ray: bilateral lower zone reticular shadowing with poorly defined diaphragms and cardiac shadows.

Lung function tests		Predicted value
$FEV_{1.0}$	1.3 litres	2.4 litres
FVC	1.5 litres	3.2 litres
Transfer factor	4 mmol/min/kPa	24 mmol/min/kPa

Questions:

1. What is the diagnosis?
2. How would you confirm this diagnosis?

Answers overleaf

48. 1. The low total T4 and free T4 indicate that the patient has become hypothyroid.

2. The TSH is probably normal because the hypothyroidism is of such recent origin that the pituitary which was previously suppressed by the hyperthyroidism has not yet responded with an increased secretion of TSH.

49. 1.(a) Primary hyperaldosteronism (Conn's Syndrome)
(b) Secondary hyperaldosteronism associated with renovascular hypertension
(c) Diuretic induced hypokalaemia

2.(a) 24 hour urine potassium excretion after discontinuing the diuretic for three days. In hyperaldosteronism the value is likely to be over 40 mmol/24 hrs whereas in diuretic induced hypokalaemia it is likely to be below 30 mmol/24 hrs.
(b) Plasma or urinary aldosterone will be high in both primary and secondary hyperaldosteronism.
(c) Plasma renin will be low in primary and high in secondary hyperaldosteronism.

50. 1. Fibrosing alveolitis
2. Lung biopsy

51. The following results were obtained in a 40 year old man six weeks after a myocardial infarction:

Serum cholesterol   12.5 mmol/l
       triglycerides   8.7 mmol/l
Lipid electrophoresis   A single broad band in the pre-beta-beta-region

Questions:

1. What disorder does he have?
2. Name two associated biochemical abnormalities.

52. A 2 month old baby has had diarrhoea and vomiting for 3 days. On admission the following results were obtained:

Plasma sodium   153 mmol/l
       potassium   4.0 mmol/l
       chloride   102 mmol/l
       bicarbonate   6 mmol/l
       urea   11.6 mmol/l
Blood glucose   20.6 mmol/l

Questions:

1. What is the cause of these abnormalities?
2. How would you treat them?
3. What two complications are likely?

Answers overleaf

51. 1. Fredrickson Type III hyperlipidaemia (Broad beta disease)
2. (a) Impaired glucose tolerance
   (b) Hyperuricaemia

52. 1. Severe dehydration. The high sodium is the result of water loss and the urea which is very high for a baby is an indication of the severity. The high blood glucose is a feature of dehydration in babies and does not indicate diabetes mellitus. The low bicarbonate is due to gastro-intestinal loss and also not to diabetes mellitus.

2. Rehydration only. Insulin should not be given.
3. Renal failure and cerebral damage.

53. A patient with pulmonary tuberculosis resistant to the standard drugs was given cycloserine and pyrazinamide. He improved clinically and radiologically but after a few weeks he became anaemic and the blood count results were as follows:

Hb 10g/dl
PVC 30%
RBC 2.8 × 10^{12}/l
MCV 106 fl
MCH 36 pg
MCHC 33%
WBC 9.0 × 10^9/l with normal differential
Platelets 210 × 10^9/l

On the blood films the RBC were reported as showing a dimorphic picture with macrocytes and target cells.

Questions:
1. What is the likely cause of the anaemia?
2. How would you prove it?
3. How would you treat it?

54. A 26 year old Indian woman who is a vegan complains of pain and weakness in her legs.

Serum calcium	1.91mmol/l
phosphate	0.9 mmol/l
alkaline phosphate	426 iu/l
albumin	42 g/l

Questions:
1. What is the most likely diagnosis?
2. What other deficiency might she have?

55. A 32 year old woman complains of breathlessness on exertion and on examination is found to be centrally cyanosed. An ear oximeter is applied and gives a reading of 57%. After breathing 100% oxygen for ten minutes, the saturation has risen to 72%.

Question:
1. What is the cause of her hypoxaemia?

Answers overleaf

53. 1. Acute sideroblastic anaemia due to cycloserine and pyrazinamide which commonly produce this complication.

2. Marrow puncture should show ring sideroblasts.
Serum B_{12} and folate concentrations are usually normal.

3. Stop the offending drugs and give pyridoxine which is usually effective.

54. 1. Osteomalacia due to dietary deficiency of vitamin D.

2.(a) Dietary deficiency of vitamin B_{12}.
This can be corrected with oral vitamin B_{12} supplements.

(b) Iron deficiency.

55. 1. An anatomical right to left shunt. All other causes of arterial oxygen desaturation will be overcome by breathing 100% oxygen.

56. An obese 52 year old business man is admitted with severe central chest pain. B.P. 140/90 mmHg.
An electrocardiogram shows an anterior myocardial infarct.

Plasma sodium	139 mmol/l
potassium	2.9 mmol/l
chloride	92 mmol/l
bicarbonate	30 mmol/l
urea	7.6 mmol/l

Question:

1. Name three types of drugs which might cause this picture.

57. A 40 year old man was admitted to hospital having been vomiting for three days. There was a history of dyspepsia but no previous respiratory problems. On examination he was dehydrated and confused. Arterial blood gases, breathing air, were as follows:

PO_2 59 mmHg (7.9 kPa)
PCO_2 64 mmHg (8.5 kPa)
pH   7.51

Questions:

1. What metabolic abnormalities do these values reveal?
2. To what is the hypoxaemia attributable?
3. Which cation will need vigorous replacement therapy to correct the metabolic abnormality?

58. A 16 year old schoolboy develops fever, sore throat and headache. On examination he has cervical lymphadenopathy and some neck rigidity.

Hb 14.8 g/dl
WBC $12.5 \times 10^9/l$
Neutrophils $3.5 \times 10^9/l$
Lymphocytes $8.5 \times 10^9/l$ of which most are atypical
ESR 20 mm/hr
CSF Lymphocytes 20/ml
Protein 0.6 g/l

Questions:

1. What is the most likely diagnosis?
2. What test would you do to confirm it?

Answers overleaf

56. 1.(a) Thiazide diuretics
   (b) Loop diuretics
   (c) Purgatives
   (d) Carbenoxolone
   (e) Corticosteroids.

57. 1. Metabolic alkalosis, probably due to pyloric stenosis following chronic peptic ulceration.

2. Hypoventilation, which is the body's defence against metabolic alkalosis, by raising PCO_2.

3. Potassium.

58. 1. Infectious mononucleosis.

In viral hepatitis, Hodgkin's disease, typhoid, brucellosis and bacterial endocarditis some atypical lymphocytes may be present but only in small numbers.

2. Paul Bunnell test which should be positive 7-10 days after the onset of symptoms.

59. A 62 year old man complained of headaches and somnolence. His arterial PCO₂ was found to be 63mmHg (8.5 kPa) at rest. Subsequent lung function tests revealed the following:

FEV 1.5 1 (50% Predicted Normal)
FVC 2.6 1 (60% Predicted Normal)

Questions:

1. What physiological abnormality does the PCO₂ reveal?
2. What is it due to?

60. A two year old boy is brought into the Accident and Emergency Department unconscious. He was perfectly well until two hours previously when he started vomiting. He is overbreathing.

Plasma sodium	129 mmol/l
potassium	3.2 mmol/l
chloride	99 mmol/l
bicarbonate	8 mmol/l
urea	7.0 mmol/l
Arterial pH	7.10
PCO₂	3.0 kPa
PO₂	11.0 kPa
Blood glucose	11 mmol/l
Urine glucose	1%, ketones trace

Questions:

1. What is the likely cause of his metabolic disturbance?
2. What biochemical investigation would you do next?

61. A 30 year old man with post-infective polyneuritis has the following values on lung function testing:

		Predicted
FEV₁.₀	2.4	4.00 litres
FVC	3.0	4.84 litres
Peak Exp. Flow Rate	285	612 1/min

Question:

1. Comment on the marked reduction in peak flow.

Answers overleaf

59. 1. Alveolar hypoventilation.

2. The reduction in ventilatory capacity is inadequate to account for this degree of hypoventilation and it must therefore be due to central (i.e. brain) insensitivity to CO_2. This can be caused by a wide variety of lesions.

60. 1. Salicylate poisoning.

In young children severe metabolic acidosis and hyperglycaemia are seen. In older children and adults respiratory alkalosis is more prominent. ·

Diabetes mellitus is unlikely in spite of the hyperglycaemia since the urine contains only a trace of ketones.

2. Plasma salicylate level.

61. 1. Disproportionate reduction in peak flow in absence of airways obstruction (normal $FEV_{1.0}$/FVC ratio) is due to muscular weakness. Peak flow is much more effort-dependant than $FEV_{1.0}$.

62. A 78 year old man is admitted unconscious after a stroke. Three days later the following results are obtained:

Plasma sodium	158 mmol/l
potassium	5.7 mmol/l
chloride	119 mmol/l
bicarbonate	23 mmol/l
urea	28 mmol/l

Questions:

1. What is the most likely cause?
2. What complication is likely to occur?

63. A 17 year old boy who had been well controlled on regular treatment for grand mal epilepsy for 10 years had recently started having more frequent fits. His medication had been increased with no beneficial effect on the fit frequency.

Serum calcium	1.8 mmol/l
phosphate	0.7 mmol/l
alkaline phosphatase	450 iu/l
folate	2 μg/l

Questions:

1. What is the likely cause for the increase in his fits?
2. What three investigations may be helpful in confirming the diagnosis?

Answers overleaf

62.   1. Dehydration due to water deprivation in an unconscious patient whose thirst mechanism is inactive.

This may be aggravated by tube feeding of a high protein, high sodium food substitute. The urea resulting from the protein breakdown and the sodium will cause an osmotic diuresis. Artificial ventilation may lead to an increase in pulmonary water loss.

2. Acute oliguric renal failure. The raised blood urea and plasma potassium may be reversible with rehydration but if the dehydration persists acute tubular necrosis will follow.

63.   1. Hypocalcaemia. The low serum calcium and phosphate and the alkaline phosphatase, which is high even for an adolescent boy, suggest that he has developed osteomalacia. The mechanism for the osteomalacia and folate deficiency described in patients on long term anticonvulsants is unclear.

2.(a) Bone X-rays.
  (b) Plasma 25-hydroxy vitamin D.
  (c) D-xylose absorption test or faecal fat estimation to exclude malabsorption.
  (d) Jejunal biopsy to exclude gluten enteropathy.

64. A 60 year old woman was admitted to hospital confused and jaundiced with a blood pressure of 95/60 mmHg. She had a cholecystectomy five years previously and had recently been taking sedatives for insomnia.

Hb	6.8g/dl
PCV	23%
MCV	71 fl
MCHC	29.6g/dl
WBC	3.1 × 10⁹/1
Serum bilirubin	90 μmol/l
alkaline phosphatase	150 iu/l
aspartate transaminase	58 iu/l
Plasma sodium	135 mmol/l
potassium	2.4 mmol/l
chloride	93 mmol/l
bicarbonate	29 mmol/l
urea	3.0 mmol/l

Questions:

1. What is the most likely cause of her clinical state?
2. Name three possible precipitating factors.

65. These are the results obtained at cardiac catheterisation of a two year old infant who had finger clubbing, cyanosis and failure to thrive.

Date	Pressures in millimetres of mercury	Oxygen saturation Percentage
SVC	—	43%
RA	10	42%
RV	120/10	43%
PA	15/5	42%
PCV (wedge)	12	98%
LA	10	88%
LV	120/8	77%
Femoral artery	120/80	75%

Questions:

1. What cardiac lesions may be present?
2. What two features would you expect to see on a plain PA chest radiograph of this infant?

Answers overleaf

64. 1. Hepatic encephalopathy.
  2.(a) Gastro-intestinal haemorrhages from oesophageal varices.
   (b) Sedatives such as barbiturates or morphine.
   (c) Diuretic therapy aggravating hypokalaemia.
   (d) Bacteraemia.

65. 1.(a) Pulmonary stenosis
   (b) Ventricular septal defect
   (c) Dextraposed aorta
  2.(a) A small pulmonary artery
   (b) Left atrium and ventricle may be small or normal in size
   (c) Hypertrophied and enlarged right ventricle producing a
    "boot-shaped" heart
   (d) Diminished lung vascularity

66. A 65 year old woman who had had backache and recurrent severe chest infections for six months develops sudden weakness of the legs and urinary retention.

Hb	6.5 g/dl
Serum calcium	3.2 mmol/l
phosphate	2.0 mmol/l
alkaline phosphatase	100 iu/l
albumin	3.0 g/l
globulin	7.1 g/l
Plasma urea	31 mmol/l

Questions:
1. What is the most likely diagnosis?
2. What two investigations would you do next?

———————————————————————

66. 1. Multiple myeloma.

The anemia is due to bone marrow infiltration. The hypercalcaemia is the result of bone destruction and the normal alkaline phosphatase indicates the absence of an osteoblastic response which is characteristic of myelomatosis. Uraemia due to obstruction of the tubiles by paraprotein may be exacerbated by renal infection, hypercalcaemia or amyloid.

2.(a) Electrophoresis of serum and urine for a monoclonal paraprotein band. Normal immunoglobulins are decreased. This depressed antibody production accounts for the infections.

(b) Bone marrow for abnormal plasma cells.

(c) Bone X-ray for characteristic circumscribed osteolytic lesions.

_____

PRACTICE EXAM — CASE HISTORIES

Candidates in the MRCP Part II examination are required to answer all 4 case histories in 55 minutes. Take this section as a mock examination and when your time is up then check your answers against the Practice Exam Answers on page 115.

1. A 65 year old woman was admitted with 10 week history of dysphagia for solids and two week history of complete dysphagia. On examination she was not icteric or pale and there were no palpable lymph glands or masses.

   Investigations:

   Hb 8.7 g/dl
   MCV 71 fl
   MCH 21 pg
   WBC 8.3 × 10⁹/1 (normal differential count)
   Platelets 200 × 10⁹/1

   Barium swallow showed complete obstruction to flow of barium in upper oesophagus.

   Oesophagoscopic biopsy revealed a squamous cell carcinoma.

   Management: she was transfused four units of packed red cells on day of admission. This raised her haemoglobin to 14.7 g/dl. She was then started on an intensive course of parenteral feeding in preparation for surgery. During this period she also received local irradiation to the tumour in a dose of 3800 rads.

   Progress: after six weeks of the above management she was found to be pancytopenic. Hb 7.5 g/dl, MCV 86 fl, MCH 27 pg, WBC 1.7 × 10⁹/1, Neutrophils 90%, Lymphocytes 10%, Platelets 10 × 10⁹/1. Liver and renal function profile normal. Bone marrow aspirate showed cellularity but no malignant cells were seen. The patient became febrile and toxic and inspite of intravenous antibiotics, died in two days.

   Questions:

   1. What is the most likely cause of the anaemia at presentation?
   2. What is the most likely cause of the pancytopenia as an inpatient?
   3. Name two specific investigations helpful to define the haematological problem.

2. A fifty three year old West Indian man was referred to an endocrine clinic with a two month history of swelling of his breast, associated with a six month history of a discharge from the right nipple. He also complained of impotence during that period with a reduced frequency of erection, inability to sustain the erection, and reduced volume of seminal fluid. He had had frequency of micturition with dysuria for four months.

He had lived in Great Britain for twenty years and his only previous history was of hypertension, diagnosed in 1974 when he had complained of headaches. He had been treated with methyldopa 250 mg twice daily since then, with control of his blood pressure. At that time he was drinking half a bottle of whisky daily and this continued for a three year period. Since that time he had reduced his alcohol intake to about 10 pints of beer a week. He was a non-smoker. He had five children and worked as a bus conductor.

On examination he had bilateral gynaecomastia with galactorrhoea from the right breast. He had normal secondary sex characteristics and external genitalia. He had a Dupuytren's contracture in the right hand. His blood pressure was 150/95 mmHg. No other abnormalities were detected.

Questions:

1. What three diagnoses would you consider to account for his signs and symptoms?
2. List five investigations you would perform.

3. A lady of 42 was admitted to hospital with a haemoptysis. There was no associated chest pain nor any shortness of breath. She was on an oral contraceptive pill. The past history included a D & C for menorrhagia some 3 years earlier. The menorrhagia had settled.

Investigations:

Haemoglobin	10.9 g/dl
WBC	$9.8 \times 10^9/1$ with 65% neutrophils
ESR	78 mm/hr

Chest X-ray showed an ill-defined opacity in the right upper zone.

Ventilation/perfusion scan showed no mismatched zones.

Subsequent course. She ceased to have haemoptysis and was very well and the chest X-ray cleared. On the day on which she was to leave hospital, the whole history was repeated but the chest X-ray now showed an ill-defined opacity in the left lower zone. Again, the symptoms cleared with clearing of the X-ray, only to recur two weeks later.

Questions:

1. Give two possible diagnoses.
2. What two investigations would you perform to confirm the diagnosis?

4. A 60 year old lorry driver gradually developed severe
generalised headaches over a period of ten days. These were
associated with nausea and intermittent drowsiness. Four days
after the onset of symptoms he had an episode of
unconsciousness lasting about 30 minutes which was not
witnessed. On the tenth day of his illness he was admitted to
hospital. On direct questioning he reported smelling a peculiar
odour occasionally since the onset of symptoms. There was no
relevant previous medical history. He smoked 60 cigarettes
daily. He was pyrexial with a temperature of 38.1°C but general
examination was otherwise normal. There was slight neck
stiffness. He was drowsy but had no focal neurological signs.
Routine heamatological and biochemical investigations were
normal, as were chest and skull X-rays. Cerebro-spinal fluid
(CSF) examination showed 120 white blood cells (60%
lymphocytes) per high power field and CSF protein was
0.8g/litre with a glucose of 3.2 mmol/litre. He was started on
intravenous ampicillin at a dose of 500 mg 6 hourly.

The next day he had a focal left-sided seizure lasting 20
minutes. On examination 24 hours later he was disorientated,
drowsy and apathetic, but his mental state fluctuated somewhat.
The optic fundi were normal. There was inattention in the left
visual fields. Tone was slightly increased in the left arm and leg
and there was mild pyramidal weakness on the left. There was
left sensory inattention. The left plantar response was extensor.
The haemoglobin was 13g/dl with a white blood cell count of
$9.0 \times 10^9/1$. Urea and electrolytes and liver function tests were
normal.

Questions:

1. Give the two most likely diagnoses.
2. List two investigations which you would do immediately.

PRACTICE EXAM — DATA INTERPRETATIONS

Candidates in the MRCP Part II examination are required to answer all 10 data interpretations in 45 minutes. Take this section as a mock examination and when your time is up check your answers against the Practice Exam Answers on page 117.

1. The following results were obtained from a cardiac catheter examination on a 45 year old man with a 12 month history of general malaise. His predominant symtoms had been dyspnoea and abdominal swelling.

    RA mean 24 mm Hg
    RV   40/24 mmHg
    LV   100/26 mm Hg
    PA (Wedge) mean 26 mm Hg

Both ventricular pressure traces showed an early diastolic dip. There was a rapid x + y descent on the right atrial pressure trace.

Questions:
1. What are the most likely diagnoses?
2. What finding on chest X-ray may help in diagnosis?

2. A 65 year old man with a long history of chest infections and breathlessness was admitted following an upper respiratory infection. On examination he was breathless, cyanosed and coughing up purulent sputum. Arterial blood gases breathing air showed:

    PCO_2 69 mmHg (9.2 kPa)
    PO_2 42 mmHg (5.6 kPa)
    pH   7.37

He was put on 28% oxygen by mask and after an hour his PO_2 and PCO_2 had become 55 and 80 mmHg respectively, with a pH of 7.32.

Questions:
1. Is his oxygenation adequate on 28% oxygen?
2. What does the increase in PCO_2 following admission indicate?
3. What is your interpretation of the pH on admission?

3. A 55 year old woman complaining of increasing tiredness was found to have an enlarged spleen without lymphadenopathy. The following results were obtained on her blood count:

Hb 9g/dl
MCV 90 fl
MCH 30 pg
MCHC 33 g/dl
WBC 45 × 10⁹/l

Differential count:

Blasts 1%
Promyelocytes 4%
Myelocytes 14%
Metamyelocytes 10%
Mature neutrophils 57%
Basophils 2%
Eosinophils 3%
Lymphocytes 6%
Monocytes 3%
Nucleated RBC 2 per 100 WBC

Questions:

1. What are the two most likely diagnoses?
2. List three further investigations that would help in differentiating between these two conditions?

4. A 19 year old male Ghanian student who has been in Britain for 2 years presents with tender cervical lymphodenopathy.

Hb 14.8 g/dl
WBC 3.4 × 10⁹/l
Differential Polymorphs 53%
Lymphocytes 17%
Turk plasma cells 23%
Platelets   normal on film
ESR 23mm/hr
Paul Bunnell   negative

Questions:

1. What is the most likely diagnosis?
2. What precautions would you advise regarding his girl friend with whom he lives?

5. A 14 year old boy being investigated for recurrent epistaxes and excessive bruising over many years gave the following results on a coagulation screen. He was not taking any drugs.

	Patient	*Control*
Prothrombin time	13 secs	12 secs
Kaolin cephalin clotting time (PTT)	60 secs	34 secs
Bleeding time	10 minutes	N = 2 to 7 minutes
Thrombin time	11 secs	11 secs

Questions:

  1. What is the likely diagnosis?
  2. List three further tests which may confirm diagnosis.
  3. How is the condition inherited?

6. The plasma from a medical student who was acting as a normal control subject was seen to be jaundiced. He was completely asymptomatic and had not taken any drugs.

Total bilirubin 48 μ mol/l
Conjugated bilirubin 15 μ mol/l
Aspartate transaminase 30 iu/l
Alkaline phosphatase 190 iu/l
Hb 15 g/dl
Reticulocytes 2%

Question:

  1. What is the diagnosis?

7. A 60 year old man with a long history of excessive alcohol consumption is admitted with severe abdominal pain.

Serum amylase 2000 iu/l
Plasma sodium 110 mmol/l
       potassium 3.0 mmol/l
       chloride 70 mmol/l
       bicarbonate 22 mmol/l
       urea 14 mmol/l
Blood glucose 10 mmol/l

The measured plasma osmolality is 280 mmol/kg and the plasma is opaque in appearance.

Question:

  1. What is the reason for his electrolyte results?

8. A 61 year old woman was admitted in a drowsy confused severely dehydrated state. Two weeks previously treatment for symptomless hypertention had been started with Navidrex K, 2 tablets daily (cyclopenthiazide with potassium chloride). At that time she had no glycosuria. Investigations on admission gave the following results:

> Blood glucose 40 mmol/l
> Plasma sodium 158 mmol/l
>   potassium 5.0 mmol/l
>   chloride 118 mmol/l
>   bicarbonate 28 mmol/l
>   urea 30 mmol/l
> Glycosuria 2%
> No ketonuria

Questions:
1. What is the diagnosis?
2. Name three groups of drugs which may precipitate this disorder.

9. A 65 year old woman with known localised Paget's disease of the right femur is seen in the Outpatients Department complaining of thirst and polyuria.

Serum calcium	3.6 mmol/l
phosphate	0.7 mmol/l
alkaline phosphatase	200 iu/l
urea	7.5 mmol/l

Questions:
1. What is the most likely cause of these results?
2. What two investigations would you do to confirm it?

10. A two week old full term fully breast fed baby has diarrhoea and convulsions.

> Blood glucose 0.5 mmol/l

Urine shows a generalised aminoaciduria and there is a positive reaction with Clinitest tablets but not with Clinistix.

Questions:
1. What is the most likely diagnosis?
2. What two tests would you do to confirm it?

PRACTICE EXAM — ANSWERS
CASE HISTORIES

1. 1. Iron deficiency.

2. Folate deficiency. The body has no long term folate stores. This patient had a reduced folate intake, during the period of her dysphagia, her carcinoma and the radiotherapy would increase folate utilisation and unless folate was specifically added she would not have received it during the period of parenteral feeding.

3.(a) Red cell folate which is the best indication of body folate status.

(b) Serum folate if red cell folate is not available.

2. 1.(a) Hyperprolactinaemia either due to a prolactinoma or secondary methyldopa therapy.

(b) Alcoholic liver disease. Skin pigmentation in a black patient makes it difficult to detect cutaneous stigmata of liver disease. However the combination of gynaecomastia, impotence and Dupuytren's contracture is suggestive.

(c) Urinary tract infection may lead to obstructive disease of the vas deferens.

(d) Diabetes mellitus

2.(a) Serum prolactin
(b) Serum testosterone
(c) Skull X-ray and pituitary fossa tomography
(d) Liver function tests including gammaglutamyltransferase
(e) MSU
(f) Intravenous pyelogram if a urinary tract infection is confirmed
(g) Urethral swab for gonorrhoea
(h) 2 hour post prandial blood glucose

3. 1.(a) Idiopathic pulmonary haemosiderosis.
If there were any evidence of glomerulonephritis the combination would suggest Goodpasture's syndrome.

(b) Wegener's granulomatosis which affects the upper or lower respiratory tract or both.

(c) Pulmonary embolism in a woman on the "pill" although the normal ventilation-perfusion scan makes this unlikely

2.(a) Pulmonary arteriogram.
(b) Lung biopsy either transbronchial or percutaneous.

4.　1.　The two most likely diagnoses are (a) cerebral abscess and (b) herpes simplex encephalitis. The development of focal neurological signs in a patient with fever and meningism warrants urgent investigation as the treatment of cerebral abscess is early surgical intervention. The course of this patient's illness would be relatively protracted for herpes simplex encephalitis. This disease may be present in a variety of ways, one of which is as a supratentorial mass lesion, particularly originating in the temporal lobe. The symptom of olfactory hallucinations in this case would be in keeping with the latter. The CSF findings would be appropriate for both diagnoses. The patient is relatively unlikely to have a cerebral tumour in the presence of fever and pleomorphic CSF and there was no obvious other systemic illness.

2.　The most important investigation is a CT head scan. This should demonstrate a cerebral abscess. In this case it showed an area of low attentuation in the right temporal lobe with oedema and shift of the mid-line structures. There was no enchancement after intravenous contrast injection, which would be expected if an abscess were present. An EEC was also performed which showed periodic complexes over the right hemisphere which are characteristically found in herpes simplex encephalitis. The EEG is also useful in the diagnosis of cerebral abscess. Typically focal high-voltage slow waves are seen. Repeat CSF examination would not yield useful diagnostic information as viral titres can only confirm herpes simplex infection retrospectively. It could be potentially dangerous if a supratentorial mass lesion is suspected, as it was here, even in the absence of papilloedema.

PRACTICE EXAM ANSWERS
DATA INTERPRETATIONS

1. 1.(a) Constrictive pericarditis.
  (b) Constrictive cardiomyopathy for example, amyloidosis.
  2. Calcification of the pericardium occurs in 50% of patients with constrictive pericarditis.

2. 1. Probably yes. A PO_2 of 55 mmHg will produce 70-80% saturation of the arterial blood.
  2. Progressive underventilation of the lungs as hypoxic drive to respiration.
  3. The normal pH with a high PCO_2 indicates a chronic, compensated respiratory acidosis.

3. 1. Myelosclerosis, chronic granulocytic leukaemia.
  2. Marrow puncture in myelosclerosis usually yields nothing or blood only and the trephine biopsy shows fibrous replacement of haematopoietic tissue. In CGL it is hyperplastic. The neutrophil alkaline phosphatase score is low in CGL and may be high, normal or low in myelosclerosis. The Philadelphia chromosome is seen in CGL and not in myelosclerosis.

4. 1. Rubella
  2. Check that she is not pregnant

5. 1. Von Willebrand's disease.
  2.(a) Factor VIII procoagulant activity.
  (b) Factor VIII antigen activity.
  (c) Platelet aggregation test with risocetin.
  (d) Platelet retention test.
  (e) Family studies.
  3. Autosomal dominant.

Von Willebrand's disease is characterised by both a vascular abnormality and platelet function defect which give rise to prolonged bleeding and also by a coagulation defect due to Factor VIII deficiency.

6. 1. Familiar unconjugated non-haemolytic hyperbilirubinaemia or Gilbert's disease.
There is a defect in the transport of bilirubin into the liver cell and in its conjugation. The condition is harmless.

7. 1. The low electrolyte results are the result of hyperlipidaemia in an alcoholic patient with acute pancreatitis. In this case the lipid is making a significant contribution to the plasma volume. Plasma electrolytes are measured in the laboratory in a given volume of fluid and if some of this fluid is lipid with a low electrolyte content, and not water, a falsely low result will be obtained.

The calculated osmolality is 250 mmol/kg which is lower than the measured osmolality and indicates that the low sodium does not indicate true hyponatraemia.

8. 1. Hyperosmolar non-ketotic diabetic coma.

This type of hyperglycaemia diabetic coma without ketonaemia or acidosis is uncommon but occurs usually in older subjects, often as the first manifestation of diabetes mellitus. When the patient recovers from the acute episode the subsequent diabetes may be very mild.

2. (a) Thiazide diuretics
   (b) Frusemide
   (c) Beta-blockers
   (d) Glucocorticosteroids

9. 1. Primary hyperparathyroidism

Hypercalcaemia of this degree is not seen in patients with Paget's disease except perhaps if they are immobilised. The low phosphate supports the diagnosis of hyperparathyroidism rather than malignancy as a cause for the hypercalcaemia

2. (a) Serum parathyroid hormone assay
   (b) Hydrocortisone suppression test

In 90% of patients with hyperparathyroidism the serum calcium remains high after hydrocortisone 150 mg daily for a week whereas in 70% of patients with hypercalcaemia due to other disorders it falls to within the normal range.

10. 1. Galactosaemia.

2. (a) Identification of urinary reducing substance as galactose by chromatography.
   (b) Red cell galactose 1—phosphate uridyl transferase activity.

CLINICAL SLIDE SECTION

In this section of the MRCP Part II examination, candidates are given approximately 2 minutes to view and answer questions related to each slide. Answers to these questions can be found on pages 151-8.

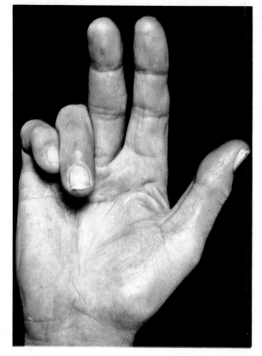

Plate 1.
1) What is this?
2) With what three conditions may it be associated?

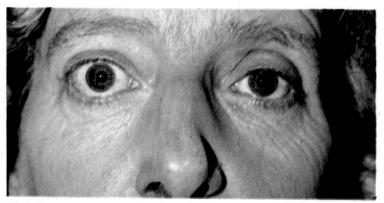

Plate 2.
1) What is the most likely cause of this?
2) Name two methods of treatment of the local lesion if it advances.

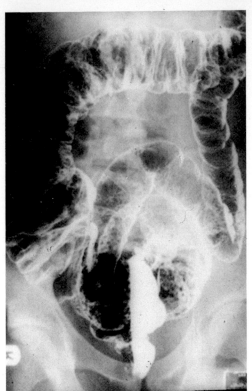

Plate 3.

1) What is the diagnosis?
2) What is the mode of inheritance?
3) What complication might arise?

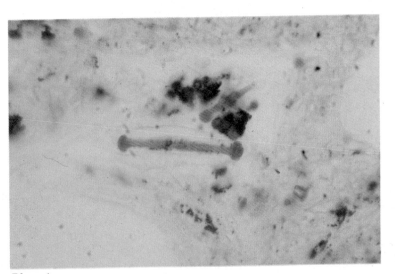

Plate 4.

1) This is an incidental finding in a patient complaining of chest pain. What is it?
2) What does it indicate?

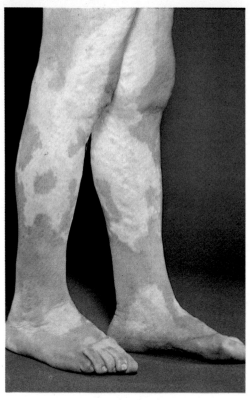

Plate 5.
1) What is this condition?
2) Name three associated conditions.

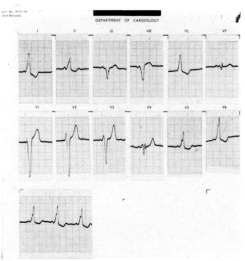

Plate 6.
1) Apart from the repolarisation abnormality, what other abnormality is seen on this ECG?
2) Name two complications.

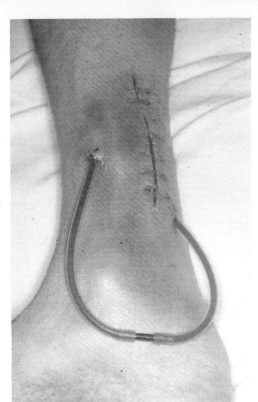

Plate 7.

1) What is this?
2) What alternative
   procedure is now
   commonly used?

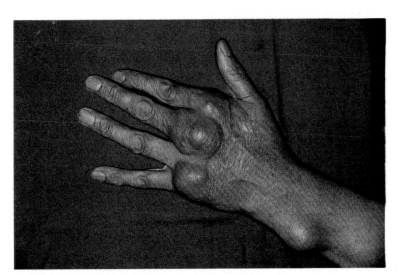

Plate 8.

1) What are these?
2) Name two complications.

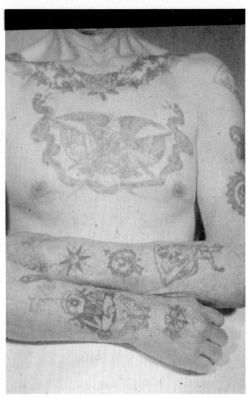

Plate 9.

1) Give three complications of this procedure.

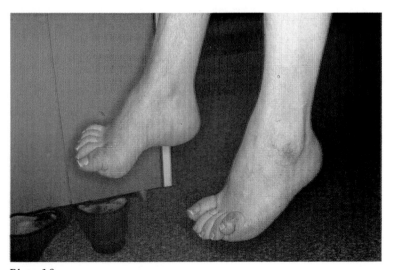

Plate 10.

1) What is this?
2) Name three causes.

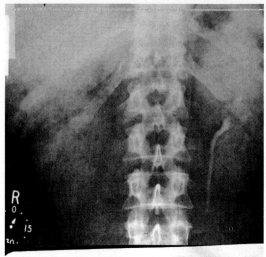

Plate 11.

1) What abnormality do these radiographs demonstrate?
2) What blood test would help in deciding on treatment?

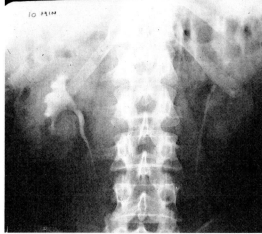

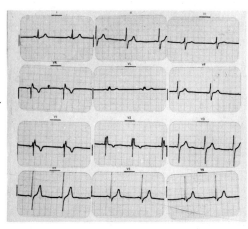

Plate 12

1) What abnormality is shown on this cardiograph of a 30 year old man?
2) What is the likely outcome?

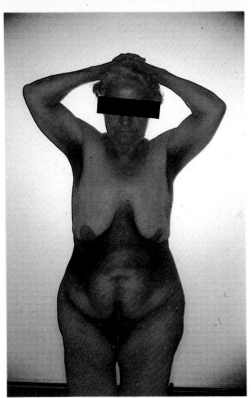

Plate 13.
1) What is this?
2) With what condition is it commonly associated?

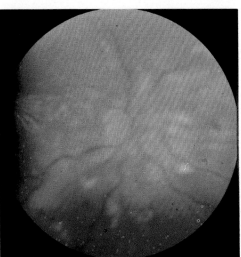

Plate 14.
1) What four abnormalities are present in this slide?
2) What is the most likely diagnosis?

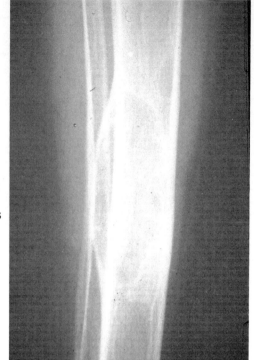

Plate 15.

1) A 43 year-old woman presented with nocturia, thirst and depression. What abnormality is shown on her X-ray?
2) What is the likely cause?

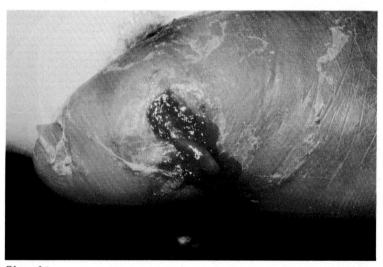

Plate 16.

1) A 33year old man developed this painless lesion after buying new shoes. What is it?
2) Give two possible causes.

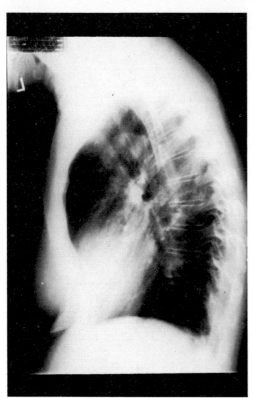

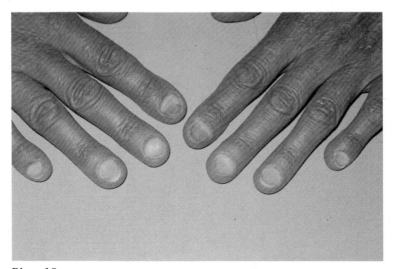

Plate 18.
1) What is this nail deformity?
2) What is the most likely cause?

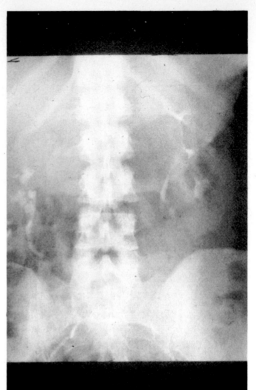

Plate 19.
1) What abnormality is shown on this urogram?
2) Give three causes.

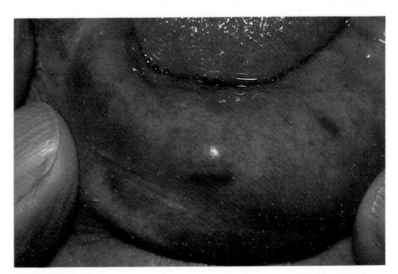

Plate 20.
1) What is the cause of this 80 year old man's gastrointestinal blood loss?
2) Give two types of treatment.

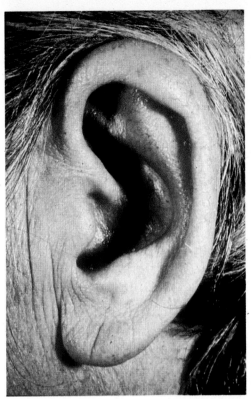

Plate 21.

1) What is the diagnosis?
2) What biochemical abnormality leads to this appearance?

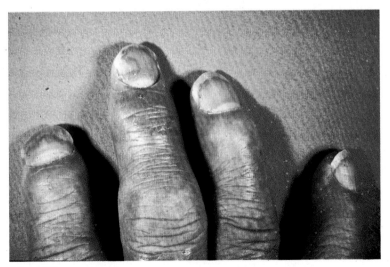

Plate 22.

1) This man presented with back pain. What is the cause of his arthropathy?
2) What joints in his back may be affected?

Plate 23.

1) What is the diagnosis?
2) What is the mode of inheritance?
3) Give three known associated disorders.

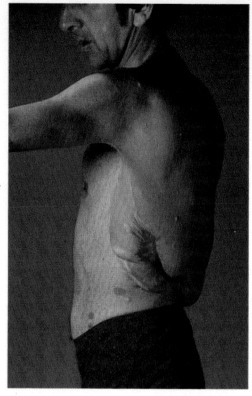

Plate 24.

1) This patient has been treated with systemic steroids for ulcerative colitis. What is the most likely cause for this chest X-ray appearance?

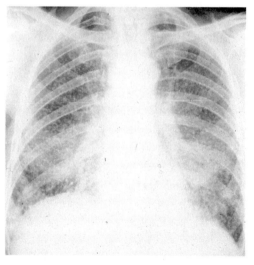

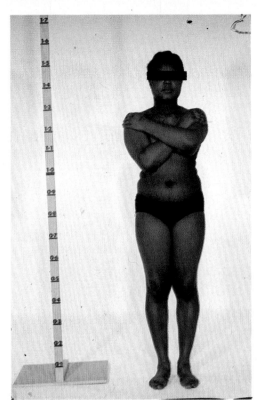

Plate 25.
1) This girl presented with secondary amenorrhoea. What is the diagnosis?
2) Give three possible causes.

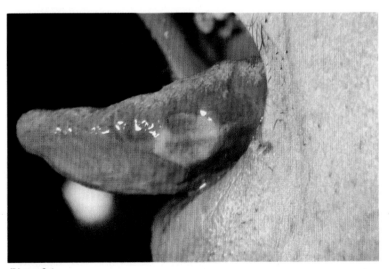

Plate 26.
1) This patient presented with a deep venous thrombosis and a painful red eye. What is the most likely diagnosis?

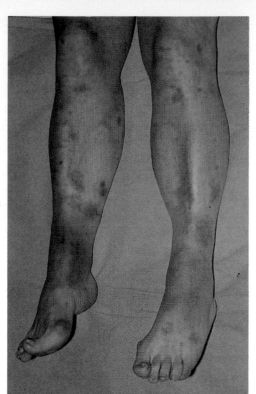

Plate 27.

1) What skin lesion is shown?
2) Give three common causes.

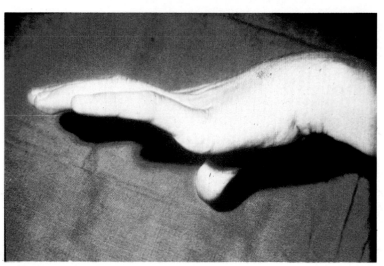

Plate 28.

1) What is the cause of this abnormality?

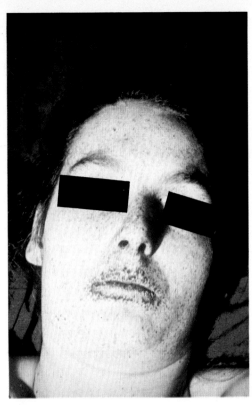

Plate 29.

1) This woman presented with intestinal obstruction. What is the diagnosis?
2) What is the likely cause of her present illness?

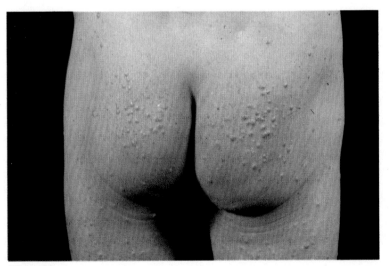

Plate 30.

1) What are the lesions shown?
2) To what three disorders may they be secondary?

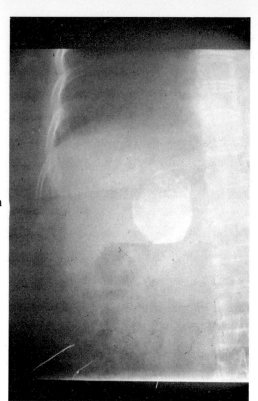

Plate 31.
1) What is the most likely diagnosis?
2) Give two tests which would help to confirm the diagnosis?

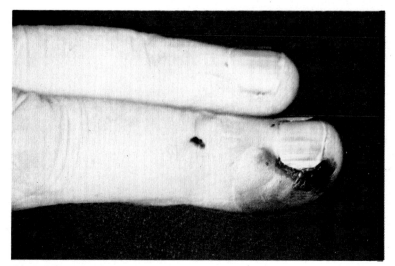

Plate 32.
1) What is this lesion?
2) What two disease processes may underly it?

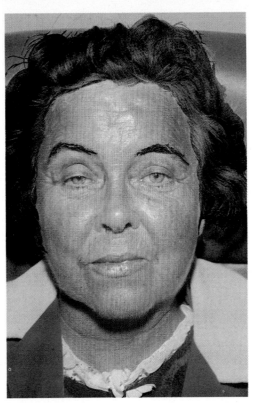

Plate 33.
1) What abnormality is shown?
2) Give three possible causes.

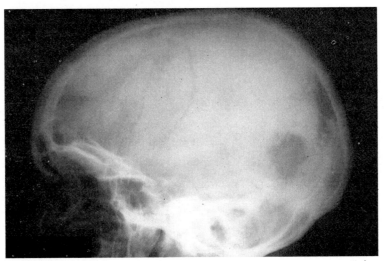

Plate 34.
1) This young man complained of polyuria and thirst. What is the likely diagnosis?
2) What is the cause of his symptoms?

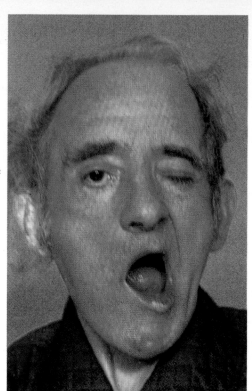

Plate 35.
1) What cranial nerve lesion does this show?
2) What evidence do you see for its cause?

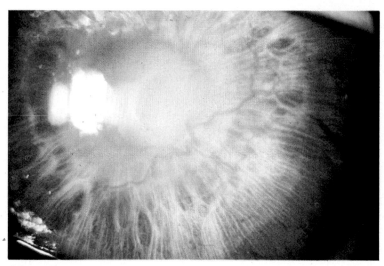

Plate 36.
1) What two abnormalities does this show?
2) What metabolic disorder could be the cause?

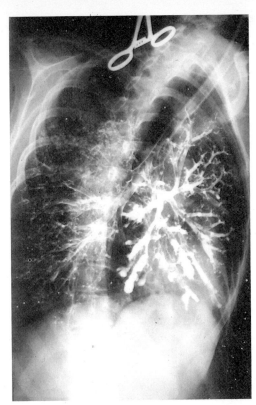

Plate 37.
1) What is the lesion shown on this chest X-ray?
2) Give three causes.

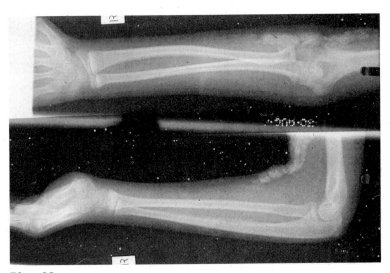

Plate 38.
1) What is the diagnosis?
2) What might you expect to see on the skin of the limb?

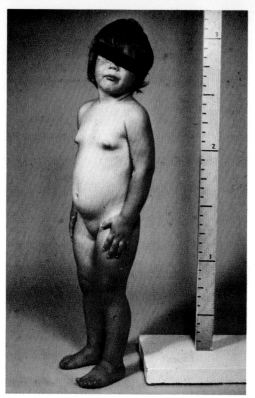

Plate 39.

1) What is the diagnosis in this 4 year old girl?
2) What two investigations in a 24 hour urine collection would be helpful in the diagnosis of the cause?

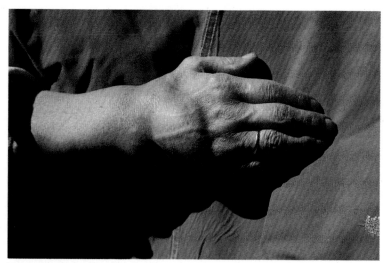

Plate 40.

1) What three abnormalities are visible on the extensor surface of this hand?
2) What is the diagnosis?

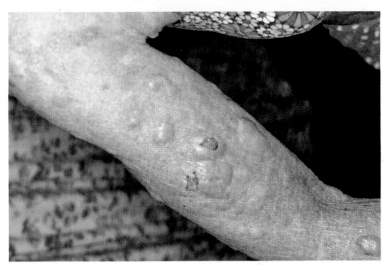

Plate 41.
1) What is the diagnosis?
2) Name three types of therapy which may be employed.

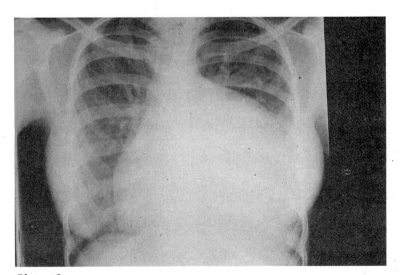

Plate 42.
1) Give two possible causes for this radiological appearance.

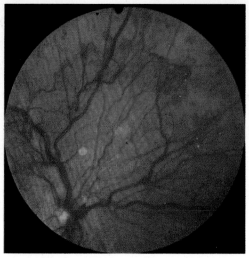

Plate 43.

1) What two abnormalities are present in this fundus?
2) What is the underlying disease?

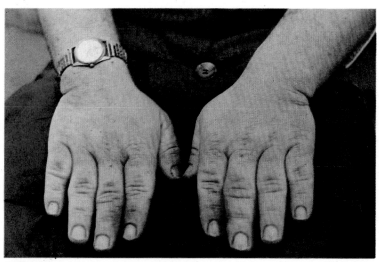

Plate 44.

1) What is the most likely diagnosis?
2) What three symptoms may the patient experience in his hands?

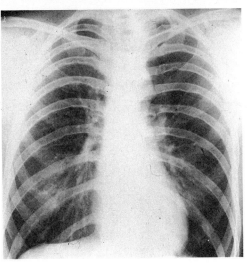

Plate 45.
1) What abnormality is shown here?
2) What three physical findings may lead to clinical detection of its cause?

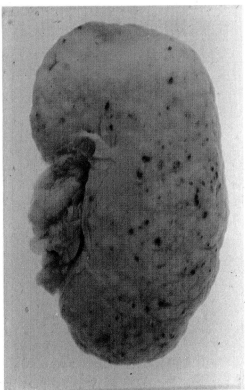

Plate 46.
1) What is the diagnosis?
2) What two abnormalities may be seen in the patient's fingers?

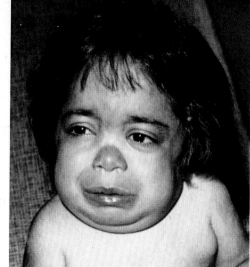

Plate 47.

1) What is the diagnosis?
2) What line of treatment may be helpful in preventing its progression?

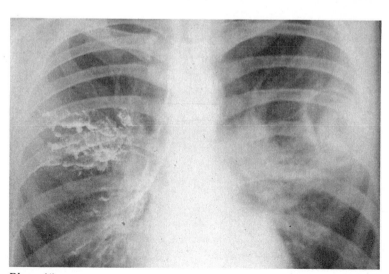

Plate 48.

1) This 16 year old boy noted a deterioration in his asthma two years ago before this X-ray. What two abnormalities does it show?

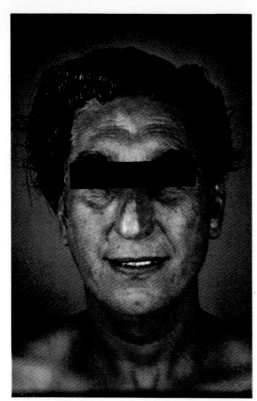

Plate 49.

1) This Englishman had an abdominal operation five years previously. What is the diagnosis?
2) What further treatment is necessary?

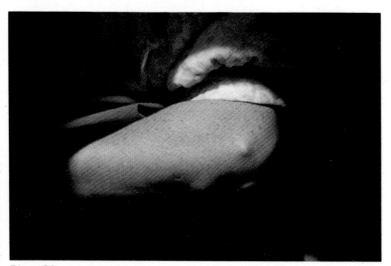

Plate 50.

1) This patient complains of symptoms suggestive of the carpal tunnel syndrome. What is the diagnosis?

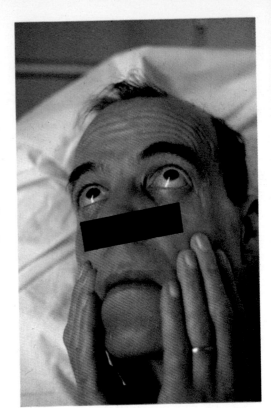

Plate 51.

1) This patient had recently been discharged from a mental hospital. Give two possible causes for his appearance.

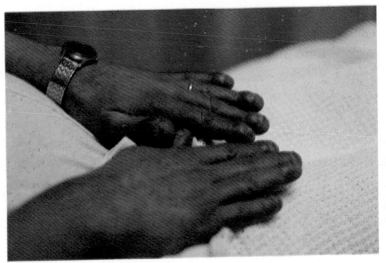

Plate 52.

1) Name five conditions which could contribute to this finding.

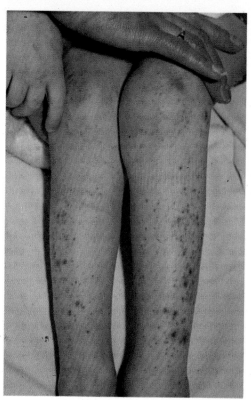

Plate 53.
1) This five year old child complained of abdominal pain. What is the probable diagnosis?
2) What three abnormalities might you find on clinical examination?

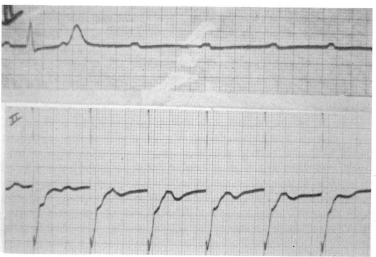

Plate 54.
1) What is the diagnosis in the upper ECG?
2) What are the changes in the lower tracing?

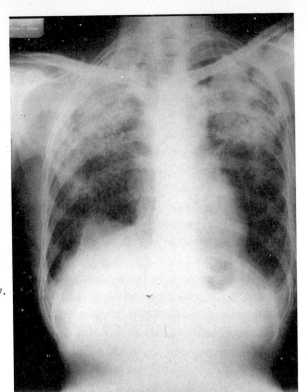

Plate 55.
1) A 40 year old coal miner attended Casualty complaining of weight loss and breathlessness over the last six months. Name two changes visible on the X-ray.
2) Give two possible causes.

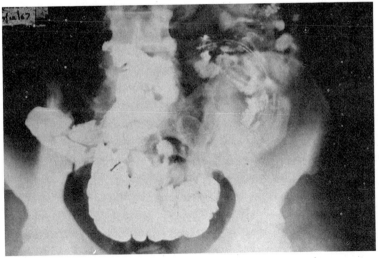

Plate 56.
1) This radiological change was an incidental finding in an African patient. Name the abnormality.
2) Give one drug used in its treatment.

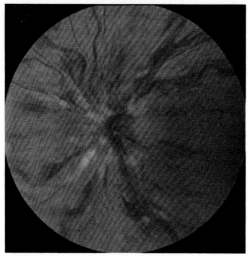

Plate 57.
1) This patient complained of loss of vision over the past two days. What two abnormalities are demonstrated?
2) What is the diagnosis?

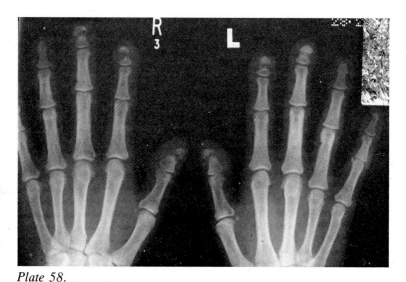

Plate 58.
1) This patient complained of nausea, constipation and polyuria. What abnoemalities are apparent on the radiograph?

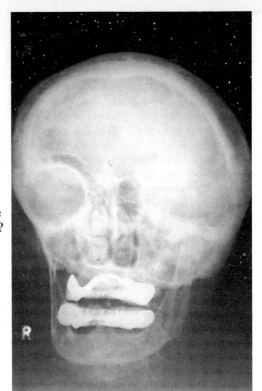

Plate 59.
1) What is the diagnosis?
2) Of what three symtoms may the patient complain?

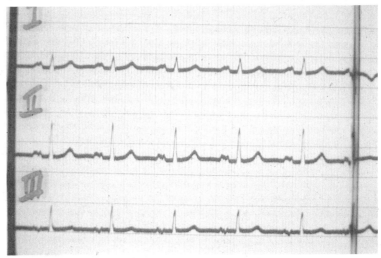

Plate 60.
1) This young man complains of breathlessness on exercise. What abnormality is apparent on the ECG?
2) What is the likely diagnosis?

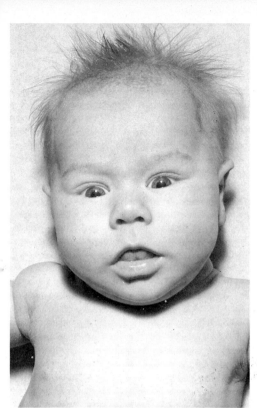

Plate 61.
1) What is the diagnosis?
2) Name three causes.

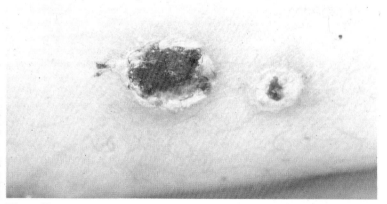

Plate 62.
1) This patient complained of periodic attacks of diarrhoea.
   What skin lesion is demonstrated?

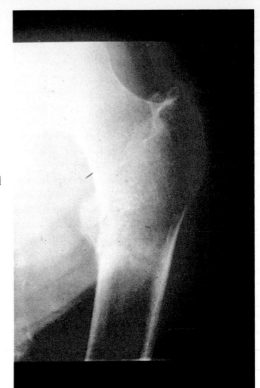

Plate 63.

1) This 23 year old woman presented with pain and weakness of the legs. What abnormality is shown on her X-ray?

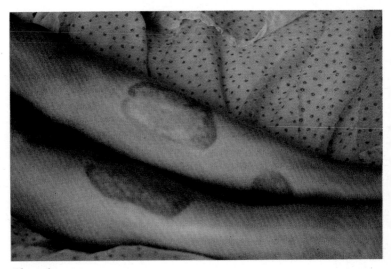

Plate 64.

1) This 43 year old lady complained of weight loss and pruritus vulvae. What is this lesion?

CLINICAL SLIDE SECTION — Answers

Plate 1.
1) Dupuytren's contracture
2) Epilepsy
   Cirrhosis—particularly alcoholic
   Chronic trauma of the hands such as that produced by long-term heavy manual work.

Plate 2.
1) Thyroid disease is the commonest cause of unilateral as well as bilateral exophthalmos.
2) Orbital decompression
   Guanethidine eye drops
   Orbital irradiation
   Intra-orbital steroids

Plate 3.
1) Multiple polyposis coli
2) Dominant
3) Carcinoma

Plate 4.
1) Asbestos body
2) Exposure to asbestos. It does not necessarily imply disease or potential disease.

Plate 5.
1) Vitiligo
2) Autoimmune thyroid disease
   Diabetes mellitus
   Pernicious anaemia
   Addison's disease
   Alopecia areata

Plate 6.
1) Wolff-Parkinson-White syndrome
2) Arrhythmias, usually supraventricular
   Sudden death

Plate 7.
1) Schribner shunt
2) Direct arterio-venous fistula

Plate 8.
1) Gouty tophi
2) Necrosis
   Secondary infection with sinus formation
   Gross joint deformity

Plate 9.

1) Serum hepatitis
   Syphilis
   Dye reaction

Plate 10.

1) Bilateral pes cavus
2) Congenital
   Friedreich's ataxia
   Poliomyelitis

Plate 11.

1) Right renal artery stenosis
2) Peripheral or renal vein renin determination
   This will help to indicate whether hypertension in such a patient is
   likely to respond to surgical correction of the stenosis.

Plate 12.

1) Partial right bundle branch block
2) A normal lifespan

Plate 13.

1) Acanthosis nigricans
2) Malignancy, for example carcinoma of the stomach or lymphoma.

Plate 14.

1) Exudates
   Haemorrhages
   Papilloedema
   Macular star
2) Grade IV hypertensive retinopathy

Plate 15.

1) Bone cyst
2) Hyperparathyroidism

Plate 16.

1) Neuropathic ulcer
2) Diabetes mellitus
   Tabes dorsalis
   Polyneuritis

Plate 17.

1) Pes excavatum   (Funnel chest)
   The depression of the lower end of the sternum causes an apparent increase in cardiac diameter on the chest X-ray which can be discounted when the narrow AP diameter is noted on the lateral view.
2) None

Plate 18.

1) Koilonychia
2) Iron deficiency

Plate 19.

1) Papillary necrosis
2) Analgesic nephropathy
   Diabetes mellitus
   Gout
   Pyelonephritis
   Sickle cell disease

Plate 20.

1) Hereditary haemorrhagic telangiectasia
2) Blood transfusion
   Oestrogens which seem to reduce the blood loss in some though not all cases.

Plate 21.

1) Alkaptonuria
2) Homogentisic acid accumulation due to deficiency of homogentisic acid oxidase. The deposits in cartilage darken. This darkening is called ochronosis.

Plate 22.

1) Psoriatic arthropathy
2) Sacro-iliac joints giving a clinical picture indistinguished from ankylosing spondylitis.

Plate 23.

1) Von Recklinghausen's disease (neurofibromatosis)
2) Dominant
3) Phaeochromocytoma
   Medullary carcinoma of thyroid
   Cystic lung disease
   Renal vascular lesions leading to hypertension

Plate 24.
1) Miliary tuberculosis

Plate 25.
1) Cushing's syndrome
2) Steroid administration
   Adrenal hyperplasia due to increased pituitary
   ACTH production
   Ectopic ACTH production
   Adrenal adenoma or carcinoma

Plate 26.
1) Behcet's syndrome
   Superficial thrombophlebitis is more usual than deep vein thrombbosis.

Plate 27.
1) Erythema nodosum
2) Streptococcal infection
   Tuberculosis
   Sarcoidosis
   Drugs

Plate 28.
1) Ulnar nerve palsy

Plate 29.
1) Peutz-Jegher syndrome
2) Intussusception of a polyp in the small intestine

Plate 30.
1) Eruptive xanthomata
2) Diabetes mellitus
   Exogenous oestrogens—e.g. the oral contraceptive pill
   Alcoholism

Plate 31.
1) Hydatid cyst of liver
2) Complement fixation test
   Haemagglutination test
   Intradermal Casoni test

Plate 32.
1) Nail-fold infact
2) Embolism—sub-acute bacterial endocarditis
   Auto-immune vasculitis—rheumatoid arthritis, systemic lupus erythematosis, polyarteritis nodosa

Plate 33.
1) Horner's syndrome
2) Apical carcinoma of the lung (Pancoast tumour)
   Cervical rib
   Syringomyelia

Plate 34.
1) Eosinophilic granuloma
2) Diabetes insipidus

Plate 35.
1) Right seventh nerve palsy (lower motor neurone)
2) Vesicles on the external auditory meatus
   The Ramsay Hunt syndrome of facial palsy and herpes zoster is due to
   involvement of geniculate ganglion of the 7th cranial nerve.

Plate 36.
1) Rubeosis iridis
   Cataract
2) Diabetes mellitus

Plate 37.
1) Bronchietasis
2) Congenital — Kartagener's syndrome
   Infections — bronchopneumonia, whooping cough, measles,
                tuberculosis, repeated infection in congenital
                agammaglobulinaemia

Plate 38.
1) Subcutaneous calcification
2) Ulceration and exudation of calcium, sclerodactyly, telangiectasiae

Plate 39.
1) Precocious puberty
2) Chorionic gonadotrophin assay—chorionepithelioma of the ovary.
   Oestrogen assay—granulosa cell or theca cell tumour or luteoma.

Plate 40.
1) Muscle wasting especially of the first dorsal interosseous
   Synovial swelling of the extensor tendon sheaths
   Synovial effusions of the metacarpophalangeal joints
2) Rheumatoid arthritis

Plate 41.

1) Mycosis fungoides
2) Topical corticosteroids in the early stages.
   Radiotherapy if the lesions are not too widespread.
   Total body electron beam therapy may produce a remission in very extensive disease.
   Photochemotherapy (PUVA) may also be effective.

Plate 42.

1) Cardiomyopathy
   Pericardial effusion
   In congestive cardiac failure with gross enlargement of the cardiac shadow Kerley's B lines in the costo-phrenic angle, which are not shown here, are seen.

Plate 43.

1) Retinal haemorrhages
   New vessel formation
2) Diabetes mellitus

Plate 44.

1) Acromegaly
2) Acroparasthesiae due to compression of the median nerve in the carpal tunnel.
   Weakness
   Pain and stiffness due to arthritis

Plate 45.

1) Rib notching
2) Hypertension
   Absent femoral pulses
   Difference in systolic blood pressure between arms (higher) and legs (lower)
   Pulsatile visible subclavian arteries
   Murmur over scapulae—site of collateral vessels
   Systolic murmur over the aortic coarctation itself

Plate 46.

1) Sub-acute bacterial endocarditis
   The typical "flea-bitten" kidney
2) Osler's nodes, splinter haemorrhages, finger clubbing

Plate 47.

1) Gargoylism
2) Bone marrow transplantation

Plate 48.

1) Aspergilloma
   Proximal bronchiectasis

Plate 49.

1) Nelson's syndrome
   Pigmentation is due to excess ACTH output and follows bilateral adrenalectomy for andrenal hyperplasia secondary to pituitary hyperplasia or pituitary adenoma.
2) Pituitary ablation surgically or by irradiation.

Plate 50.

1) Rheumatoid arthritis
   This is a rheumatoid nodule.

Plate 51.

1) Jaundice due to a phenothiazine drug such as chlorpromazine
   Infective hepatitis which may spread through institutions such as mental hospitals.

Plate 52.

1) Cyanotic congenital heart disease
   Pulmonary fibrosis
   Sub-acute bacterial endocarditis
   Suppurative lung disease
   Hepatic cirrhosis
   Ulcerative colitis
   Crohn's disease

Plate 53.

1) Henoch-Schönlein purpura
2) Hypertension
   Oedema
   Joint tenderness

Plate 54.

1) Complete heart block
2) Ventricular pacing

Plate 55.

1) Bilateral upper lobe fibrosis
   Cavitation
   Tenting of the right diaphragm
2) Progressive massive fibrosis
   Tuberculosis

Plate 56.
1) Ascaris lumbricoides
2) Piperazine

Plate 57.
1) Engorged retinal veins
   Haemorrhages
2) Central retinal vein thrombosis

Plate 58.
1) Collapse of terminal phalanges of both thumbs index and middle
   fingers. Soft tissue "pseudo-clubbing" is apparent.

Plate 59.
1) Paget's disease
2) Increase in size of the head
   Headaches
   Tinnitus
   Vertigo
   Hearing loss

Plate 60.
1) Bifid P waves
2) Mitral stenosis

Plate 61.
1) Congenital hypothyroidism (cretinism)
2) Thyroid dysgenesis or rarely agenesis
   TSH deficiency
   Inborn deficiency of one of the enzymes of thyroid
      hormone synthesis.

Plate 62.
1) Pyoderma gangrenosa in a patient with ulcerative colitis

Plate 63.
1) Looser zone or pseudo-fracture
   which is diagnostic of osteomalacia

Plate 64.
1) Necrobiosis lipoidica diabeticorum